YOUR
CHILD'S
F O O D
ALLERGIES

Other Wiley Health Titles

No More Sleepless Nights, Peter Hauri, PhD and Shirley Linde, PhD

Alzheimer's: A Caregiver's Guide and Sourcebook, Howard Gruetzner

The 50+ Wellness Program, Harris H. McIlwain, Lori F. Steinmeyer, Debra Fulghum Bruce, R. E. Fulghum, Robert G. Bruce, Jr.

The Family Genetic Sourcebook, Benjamin A. Pierce

Diabetes: The Facts That Let You Regain Control of Your Life, Charles Kilo, MD and Joseph R. Williamson, MD

The Chronic Bronchitis and Emphysema Handbook, Dr. François Haas and Dr. Sheila Sperber Haas

Osteoporosis, Harris H. McIlwain, Debra Fulghum Bruce, Joel C. Silverfield, Michael C. Burnette

Caring for Your Own: Nursing the Ill at Home, Darla N. Neidrick, RN

Medical Botany: Plants Affecting Man's Health, Walker H. Lewis and Memory P. F. Elvin-Lewis

Quick Medical Terminology: A Self-Teaching Guide 3rd Edition, Genevieve Love Smith, Phyllis E. Davis, Shirley S. Steiner

Winning With Arthritis, Harris H. McIlwain, MD, Joel C. Silverfield, MD, Michael C. Burnette, MD, Debra Fulghum Bruce.

The No-Hysterectomy Option: Your Body—Your Choice, Herbert A. Goldfarb, MD, with Judith Greif, MS, RNC

Your Premature Baby: Everything you need to know about the Childbirth, Treatment, and Parenting of Premature Infants, Frank P. Manginello, MD and Theresa Foy DiGeronimo, MEd

Living Well with Parkinsons: An Inspirational, Informative Guide for Parkinsonians and Their Loved Ones, Glenna Wotton Atwood with Lila Green Hunnewell.

The BackPower Program, David Imrie, MD and Lu Barbuto, DC

The Foot Book: Lifetime Relief for Your Aching Feet, Glenn Copeland, DPM with Stan Soloman

YOUR
CHILD'S
FOOD
ALLERGIES

Detecting & Treating Hyperactivity, Congestion, Irritability and other Symptoms Caused by Common Food Allergies

JANE McNICOL

John Wiley & Sons, Inc.
New York • Chichester • Brisbane • Toronto • Singapore

LIBRARY OF CONGRESS CATALOGING IN PUBLICATION DATA

McNichol, Jane.
    Your child's food allergies : detecting & treating hyperactivity, congestion, irritability, and other symptoms caused by common food allergies / by Jane McNicol.
      p. cm.
    Includes bibliographical references and indexes.
    ISBN 0-471-55801-X (pbk.)
    1. Food allergy in children—Popular works.   I. Title.
RJ386.5.M37   1992
618.92'97'5—dc20   91-34661

Printed and bound by Courier Companies, Inc.

*To all parents of very active, inattentive children —
commonly referred to as "hyperactive." If food is one of the
culprits contributing to your child's daily miseries, this book
will help you solve the diet puzzle.*

CONTENTS

ACKNOWLEDGMENTS

MANY PEOPLE and groups have made this project possible and have contributed to our knowledge of the relationship between diet and hyperactivity.

Initially, in 1978, Helen Dadiotis, RD, then director of dietetics at Alberta Children's Hospital, encouraged me to explore the effect of diet on behavior and to do clinical work in this area. Sharon Tateishi, RD, and Nancy Lundhild, RD, offered technical support, backup, advice and encouragement. They made themselves available for several years. During the three years it took to collect data for research, the staff from the Department of Dietetics tested recipes, prepared food for research families and never complained about changed schedules, overtime and more than a few frustrating moments.

In 1981, a research team was assembled to evaluate prior research and my clinical work and to develop a research proposal. We have now worked together for more than eight years and hope to conduct more studies on the effect of diet on behavior in the future. The other members of the team are: Bonnie J. Kaplan, PhD, Department of Pediatrics and Psychology, University of Calgary and Alberta Children's Hospital Research Centre; Richard A. Conte, PhD, The Learning Centre, and Department of Psychology, University of Calgary; and H.K. Moghadam, MD, Department of Pediatrics, University of Calgary and Alberta Children's Hospital. Dr. Kaplan, who continues to write and present seminars on this topic, is becoming known as an international expert on diet and hyperactivity. Her staff at the Research Centre provides us with ongoing support.

Many other departments at Alberta Children's Hospital provided reports, information, discussion and support; just to name a few—the developmental clinics, the departments of psychology, social work and preschool. Deserving a special mention for their contribution are Jim Winning, MSW, and Kathy McFee, MSW, two innovative social workers who developed and conducted a marvelous parent support program for families of hyperactive children. Special thanks go to psychologist Jim Bannard, who is very knowledgeable about hyperactivity. Jim was my first professional contact in the field. He patiently taught me how to put diet and hyperactivity into perspective and how to deal with stressed families, and I still consult him.

In addition to the professional staff and volunteers at Alberta Children's Hospital, many others have contributed greatly, including: the Calgary Association for Children and Adults with Learning Disabilities, especially member Sue Jennings; and Phyllis Kane, founder of the Allergy Asthma Association of Calgary. I shall be forever indebted to the Allergy Information Association of Canada for its advice and the wonderful educational material developed by its tireless executive director, Susan Daglish.

Some of the recipes in this book have been adapted from other sources. The majority were developed by the parents of hyperactive children and dietitians at Alberta Children's Hospital. I would like to acknowledge two books and authors in particular: *The Taming of the Candy Monster* by Vicky Lansky and *Feeding Your Child* by Louise Lambert-Lagacé.

Finally, I am grateful to the hundreds of parents and children who were referred for research and for clinical counseling. They have provided the hands-on experience and dialogue. Each one has made a very valuable contribution.

YOUR
CHILD'S
FOOD
ALLERGIES

Introduction

We were just about to say that nothing was changing (and why were we eating this way) when our daughter started sleeping through the night! Almost four years old! With the needed sleep, she became the little girl we always knew was in there! Not perfect, but so much happier, with more energy and able to listen and try things for herself! A more normal little girl!

—MOTHER OF A THREE-YEAR-OLD UNDERACTIVE GIRL WHO SLEPT POORLY AND HAD A POOR ATTENTION SPAN

In 1978, THE ADMINISTRATION at Alberta Children's Hospital in Canada agreed to have the Department of Dietetics counsel families with hyperactive children. During the next eight years, approximately 800 families were provided with this service. All families were referred by their physicians. Initially, the diet used in the program was based on information which suggested that artificial colors, flavors and foods high in salicylates (aspirin-like compounds which occur naturally in many fruits, vegetables, herbs, spices and nuts and artificially in many medications) could have adverse effects on hyperactive children and should therefore be restricted from their diet. One of the many advocates of this belief was Dr. Ben Feingold, author of *Why Your Child Is Hyperactive*. In accordance with his suggestion, we removed foods which were considered to be high in salicylates from the diet. Over the course of our study, however, we came to

1

suspect that only a small percentage of the children were intolerant of all foods high in salicylates. Instead, they appeared to be intolerant of foods containing naturally occuring salicylates to which they had been frequently exposed—foods such as, apples, oranges, tomatoes, corn, grapes and raisins. We also observed that children who had been fed large amounts of juice as babies, due to cow's milk and infant formula intolerance, later developed intolerances to them.

It soon became apparent that the youngsters participating in the diet were reacting to all sorts of different combinations of foods and chemicals not previously considered to cause behavior problems. Among the offending foods were: milk and dairy products and chocolate. The children also reacted to other substances such as excessive simple sugars; caffeine-containing products; monosodium glutamate and its kissing cousins, hydrolyzed vegetable protein and hydrolyzed plant protein. However, they reacted less frequently to these substances than to the first three allergens. Some children also reacted to food preservatives.

One conclusion that was evident was that no two children reacted to exactly the same combination of items in the same way. Each child's reaction was unique.

The development of our Hyperactivity Test Diet at Alberta Children's Hospital was unique in one respect. Many of the referrals were from developmental clinics, departments of social work and psychology, and pre-school programs evaluating youngsters for school placement. Many of the professionals involved in these programs were extremely interested in the experimental work being done with diet at the hospital and were willing to share their ideas about the effects of diet on their young charges. Their knowledge and assessments also helped to determine not only areas in which diet could be effective but also the areas not altered by diet.

By 1981, enough interest had been generated in this

work to assemble a research team. The team was led by Dr. Bonnie Kaplan, the director of the Behavioral Research Unit at Alberta Children's Hospital, and included two other research psychologists, a pediatrician with a developmental specialty and myself. Together we developed a proposal to determine if any aspect of diet, food allergy, intolerance or nutrient intake affected the behavior, sleep or physical symptoms of twenty-four preschool boys diagnosed as hyperactive. In January 1983, funding was granted by the Alberta Mental Health Research Advisory Council and the National Health Research and Development Program of Health and Welfare Canada.

Our first families began the diet in the spring of 1983. After extensive screening, they were taught to weigh and measure all food to be eaten by the hyperactive child and to keep detailed diaries, noting their child's sleep and behavior problems and physical symptoms. For three weeks they kept their records and fed their families as they had previously. For the next seven weeks similar records were kept, but food for the entire family was provided by the hospital. All labels and tell-tale packaging were removed. Much of the food was prepared by the hospital kitchen staff. Several local food producers cooperated and prepared such items as additive-restricted bakery products, deli meats and uncolored butter. Many hospital volunteers shopped for unusual items, repackaged foods and helped with accounting and the many other mechanics involved in a project of this complexity.

For three weeks the families received foods similar in brands and nutrients to those they had received during the first three weeks. For four weeks they received foods containing no artificial colors or flavors and low in simple sugars (table sugar, syrups and honey). In addition, foods containing sugar were distributed over six feedings. Caffeine, including chocolate, was eliminated, as was monosodium glutamate and related substances. Although it has been suggested that nitrates may affect behavior, we decided to include specially prepared deli meats preserved with minimal amounts of nitrates (wieners, ham, bacon and a luncheon meat somewhat like bologna) in order to make the test diets as much like the children's normal diets as possible. As well, many highly nutritious foods, such as beets, spinach and broccoli, which are high in nitrates, were not excluded. The food preservatives butylated hydroxytoluene (BHT) and butylated hydroxyanisole (BHA) were eliminated. The preservatives benzoic acid and sodium benzoate were restricted. However, benzoates that occur naturally in foods such as prunes, berries, cinnamon and anise were not removed from the diet.

If the child's individual assessment indicated that he or she was intolerant of other foods, they were removed as well. Milk and dairy products were removed from some children's diets, while oranges, apples, grapes, raisins, tomatoes and/or corn were removed from others'. Only a few of the children were on a salicylate-restricted diet. As in my clinical practice, less than 20 percent of the children appeared to be in need of salicylate restriction.

Data collection for the diet was completed in May of 1986. It took three years to complete the experiment as each of the twenty-four families participated in the diet in succession rather than all at once.

There was one very important factor affecting the results of this study. At the end of the project, none of the parents was able to tell the research team what dietary measures were taken or when they had been in the diet phase. They had been led to believe that different foods and additives were constantly being experimented with every day or every few days. It was extremely important that the parents be unaware of our design so that the observations they recorded in their diaries about their children's behavior, sleep patterns and physical symptoms were unbiased.

In the end, the results of this study showed that the behavior of over half the children had improved while they were on the diet. In most cases, their sleep patterns had also improved and their physical symptoms had subsided.

CHAPTER ONE

Food And The Hyperactive Kid

*As an infant, our youngest child of three (now four years old)
had lots of diarrhea and stomachaches, which we linked to food
sensitivities. When his diarrhea disappeared, we thought he had
outgrown his allergies. However, he was an overly challenging
and unhappy child. He was very impatient, got easily upset,
cried a lot and constantly pushed limits to extremes.*
—MOTHER OF A FOUR-YEAR-OLD HYPERACTIVE BOY

PARENTING JUST ISN'T WHAT it is cracked up to be
when you find that you have a hyperactive child. Unlike
most other childhood disorders, little has been known or
understood about the many causes of hyperactivity, also
called Attention Deficit Disorder with Hyperactivity
(ADDH) by the medical profession.

My favorite medical expert and co-researcher on hyperactivity, Dr. Joe Moghadam, recently published a book
on hyperactivity called *Attention Deficit Disorder: Hyperactivity Revisited.* In his book, he describes hyperactivity as
a disorder consisting of chronic inattention, impulsivity,
purposelessness, overactivity, difficulties of social inter-
action and a number of associated symptoms. He reports
prevalence of hyperactivity in 2 to 3 percent of girls and
in 6 to 9 percent of boys in the United States, Great
Britain, Australia, Germany and China, with higher rates
in Italy, Spain and New Zealand.

There is no one known cause of hyperactivity, and

often no specific cause can be found. Some suspected causes include inappropriate or inadequate parenting or schooling, and stress-producing situations in the home or at school. Among other possible causes are: brain damage or malfunction; genetic influences such as a family history of hyperactivity; birth complications; epilepsy; atopic diseases such as eczema and asthma; chromosomal abnormalities; metabolic disorders; social or emotional immaturity. It is also believed that environmental poisoning, including lead poisoning, can lead to hyperactivity as, quite possibly, can prenatal smoking, alcohol use and drug use or abuse during pregnancy. Food allergy and intolerance of food additives—the main areas of interest in our study—can also cause hyperactivity.

Hyperactivity caused by food intolerance seems to have been much less prevalent before World War II than it is now. In those days, breakfast consisted of oatmeal or an egg and toast. Bread was purchased one loaf at a time. It quickly became moldy in the days before the addition of preservatives. During World War II, money was scarce, leaving little extra for special foods. Store-bought ice cream was considered a great treat. Since refrigerators were rare, having ice cream for dessert meant making a quick trip to the pharmacy at the end of the main course. Refrigerators, if you were lucky enough to have one, lacked freezer space, so there were no readily available Dingdongs, Ice Pops, Eskimo Pies and so on, which children now consider commonplace. There was no television, let alone TV dinners. The Golden Arches and other fast food franchises had not yet appeared. Food manufacturers, especially the cereal producers, were by today's standards unimaginative: no colors, no flavors, no chocolate, no marshmallows, no sugar, no preservatives. As many of my young friends would say, "Boring!" As well, we were deprived of sugary powdered drinks because they simply didn't exist. Crayons, pencils, erasers and gold stars were the tools of our trade at school.

Magic markers, whiteout, smelly stickers and room deodorizers had not yet made their appearance.

There must have been hyperactive children back then. Perhaps they were given a different label, but they certainly were not as numerous or as visible as they are now according to many older teachers. Nor did there appear to be nearly as many allergic children as there are today. One possible explanation for this could be the fact that most of the advances in the treatment of allergic disease have occurred in the past thirty years. Before then, most allergic children either died young or were too ill to attend school. With the advances in modern medicine, many severely allergic people are now leading normal productive and reproductive lives. Because there is definitely an inherited tendency to be allergic, these allergic parents will pass on the tendency to their children, and more of that generation will survive long enough to pass it on to their children, thus creating more allergic people.

With the incidence of food intolerance and hyperactivity on the rise, the need for finding ways of treating these conditions becomes all the more critical.

CHAPTER TWO

THE TREATMENT QUAGMIRE

I can accept behavior management counseling, but drugs scare me half to death. Tell me that diet is the answer.
—MOTHER OF A SIX-YEAR-OLD HYPERACTIVE BOY

NEXT TO COPING WITH the hyperactive child, often a parent's greatest frustration is dealing with the medical community and its bewildering opinions on how best to treat the child.

Behavior management training and medication of one sort or another are the two most common physician-prescribed therapies.

BEHAVIOR MANAGEMENT TRAINING

BEHAVIOR MANAGEMENT TECHNIQUES are often helpful in coping with hyperactive children. The hyperactive child is caught in a vicious circle. Perhaps because of a food intolerance, he's hyperactive. But because of his hyperactivity, he does not develop proper social skills and creates many family problems and arguments. This only increases his tendency to act out.

Teaching the child how to cope socially can reduce the tension-producing hyperactivity.

DRUG THERAPY

YOU SHOULD ALSO consider drug therapy. The most frequently prescribed medication for hyperactive children is methylphenidate (Ritalin). Its use has increased dramatically in recent years, which has sparked concern among parents, who fear overuse or misuse. But Ritalin, when appropriately prescribed and monitored by a pediatrician, can be of tremendous value. It works wonders for some children, as it improves concentration and fine motor skills. One warning: it is better to use 10 mg tablets than 20 mg ones. The latter contain tartrazine (yellow dye #5), which some children react to; the 10 mg tablets are free of the dye.

One advantage to Ritalin is that it can be used in conjunction with a diet trial. The drug does not specifically relieve allergies, allergy-caused physical symptoms or sleep disturbances, so dietary progress can be monitored in these areas. Furthermore, some children respond well to Ritalin and not to dietary changes.

FOOD ALLERGY TESTING

DIETARY TREATMENT of hyperactivity is even more controversial than drug therapy. Part of the problem is proper diagnosis of food allergies. Traditionally, if a parent and physician suspect that a child is allergic to different foods, the allergist will order allergy testing, the most common being the scratch test.

In this test, the allergist places on the skin an extract made from the allergen, and then scratches the area with a needle. If the area reddens or swells, the test is considered positive, indicating an allergy. Many physicians are reluctant to perform scratch tests on infants and young children because it irritates their skin and may frighten them. Furthermore, these tests tend not to be very accurate when used alone. It is more effective to use them in conjunction with food elimination trials.

Another frequently used test is called RAST (radioallergosorbant) testing. Blood is drawn and tested for food allergies. This test is probably not any more accurate than scratch testing, and it is very expensive.

There are other tests for food allergy, but most are not considered valid by traditional medical people. These include cytotoxic, intracutaneous and sublingual testing. In my experience, traditional allergy testing (scratch and RAST) results have been more useful in isolating problem foods than these other methods of testing.

Some physicians prefer to put their young charges on elimination diets, removing the most common food allergens, such as milk, chocolate, egg, corn, wheat and soy, to determine just what might be the culprit. The doctor will suggest the parent eliminate the offending food from the child's diet long enough to determine whether abnormal behavior, or more commonly, eczema, asthma, runny nose—or whatever other symptoms there may be—are thereby relieved.

Other doctors use allergy tests to determine more specifically what should be eliminated.

Adding to the problem of accurate diagnosis is the fact that there are two other categories of food intolerance that may affect a child's behavior. The first is *non-allergic food intolerance* and the second is *psychological intolerance.*

Non-Allergic Food Intolerance

It is more than a little frustrating to parents to be told, perhaps after allergy testing and elimination diets, that their child's explicit behavioral reactions to foods or drugs are not caused by allergies. What the doctor may not have explained clearly is that there are reactions to food that are not associated with allergies per se, that is with the immune system response. Some examples: caffeine jitters and irritability, monosodium glutamate-induced headaches, migraines brought on by specific proteins (tyramines) and behavioral responses to salicylates. It has been reported that most behavioral reactions to artificial colors and flavors are not immune-system mediated.

To repeat: discomfort caused by various foods does not

always indicate a food allergy. This does not mean the discomfort is any the less real or problematic. Many people are bothered by milk. They are not allergic to milk, but they certainly learn to avoid it if they also want to avoid upset stomachs and diarrhea.

PSYCHOLOGICAL INTOLERANCES

SOME REACTIONS TO FOODS may be categorized as psychological intolerances, in which food is associated with a bad experience. Has this ever happened to you? You are in a restaurant. The waiter brings you a perfectly cooked leg of lamb, but as you are about to take your first bite, a cockroach peeks out from under the parsley garnish. You stand a good chance of reacting—not allergically, but psychologically—to the next leg of lamb you are served!

This happens with children, too. For example, a child has a big bowl of chili for dinner and later that evening comes down with a bad case of the stomach flu. Not surprisingly, he subsequently develops an aversion to chili.

Perhaps I have not helped you out of the treatment quagmire. The best thing is to try a variety of methods, even in combination with each other. For instance, Ritalin in association with behavior management training may clear up hyperactivity and indicate that food is not the problem. But what if hyperactivity continues, perhaps associated with other reactions, such as asthma? Then Ritalin and/or counseling may alleviate hyperactivity just enough to allow you to concentrate on what foods might be causing the problem.

Allergy tests and elimination diets might then be the next step in resolving your dilemma.

Keep your options open. Be patient as you consult various experts. Explore all possibilities—and read on, for this book may be the best help for you yet!

Is Your Child A Good Candidate For The Diet?

Katie was a little girl who did not seem very happy, cried a lot, slept very poorly, had little energy. Our biggest concern, however, was fits of uncontrollable laughter and becoming so awkward she would fall down as if she had been drinking. We finally saw these as occurring just after eating. It was such a sudden and dramatic change from lethargy to hyperactivity.
—PARENTS OF A THREE-YEAR-OLD GIRL WHO ALTERNATED BETWEEN HYPOACTIVITY AND HYPERACTIVITY

BEFORE BECOMING INVOLVED in the Hyperactivity Test Diet you should discuss it with your family physician. You will need your doctor's support in determining that your child is healthy and that his or her abnormal behavior is not likely to be a result of a physical illness and/or social problems. It would be a shame if more pressing treatment were delayed by a diet trial.

Generally, the children who have responded well to a diet trial are those who come from a family with a history of food and/or environmental allergy and food intolerance. They are often balky, picky, poor eaters. As parents, you can help to determine whether a diet trial will benefit your child by examining your own reactions to food.

PARENTS' QUESTIONNAIRE

- Are you adversely affected by food?
- Does sugar make you sleepy or more active?
- Does caffeine make you jittery, affect your sleep or upset your stomach?
- Do baked beans, onions or cucumber make you gassy?
- Do you get rashes or hives after eating strawberries or tomatoes?
- Does red wine or old cheese trigger a migraine?
- Do you get irritable, jumpy, grumpy or develop a headache if you don't eat for several hours?
- Do you get wheezy, full of mucus or develop a headache, stomachache or diarrhea when you drink cow's milk?
- Do you develop a headache, tightness in the chest or tingling in the mouth when you have Chinese food or eat foods laced with monosodium glutamate?
- Do you suspect that you react to foods containing artificial sweeteners with headaches, bloating or stomachaches?
- Do you crave and/or binge on certain foods such as cola, chocolate or even alcohol?
- Do you get rashes or itchy skin from certain soaps, aftershaves, cosmetics or detergents?
- Do you get headaches, nausea or become irritable when you are exposed to certain perfumes or cleaning supplies?
- Do certain pollens or dust give you hay fever?
- Do markers, whiteout or nail polish remover make you light-headed, give you headaches, or do you just love the smell of them?
- Do aerosols and cigarette smoke make it difficult for you breathe?

If your answer is yes to two or more of these questions, how great is your ability to concentrate, to sleep or to be pleasant when you have these symptoms? As an adult, you are much more likely to be able to put a lid on your reactions than a small child suffering from quite similar symptoms.

The following list of indicators was developed to give health professionals and teachers a tool to quickly identify youngsters who might respond to a diet trial, and may also help you decide whether your child is a good prospect for this diet plan. Although it was originally designed for four-to six-year-olds, it can be used for children of all ages.

KEY INDICATORS FOR DIET TRIAL

• Child has trouble falling asleep at night.
• Child awakens during the night.
• Child gets up during the night.
• Child frequently has bad breath.
• Child frequently has a stuffy or runny nose.
• Child frequently is on or has been on medications.
• Child has unusual reactions to medications, especially to those which are artificially colored and flavored.
• Child has been allergic to or intolerant of foods or formula in infancy.
• Child has had noticeable reactions to specific foods.
• Parent is allergic to, intolerant of or dislikes cow's milk.
• Mother had multiple food cravings and/or aversions to certain foods during pregnancy.
• Father or mother is intolerant of caffeine or has a very limited tolerance for it.
• There is a family background of food allergy, food intol-

erance, environmental sensitivity or food-triggered migraine.

Sleep disturbances and frequent use of medications are common to many disorders, but if you have answered yes to one or more of the other questions, a diet trial could be worthwhile.

At least 20 percent of the children referred for this type of counseling are adopted. In most cases little is known of the birth parents' backgrounds. Parents with adopted youngsters will be gambling a little more in making their decision, but it can be based solely on their observations of the child's reactions to foods, behavior, sleep problems and physical symptoms.

CHAPTER FOUR

WHAT YOUR CHILD WILL EAT ON THE DIET

For a mother and father who were not used to cooking and baking a lot, it was a change for us. But after a while on the diet we have become more careful shoppers and have discovered new things. It is not a restricted diet in the sense that you have little variety, and it's probably opened our family up to eating a wider, better balanced variety of foods.

—FATHER OF A FOUR-YEAR-OLD HYPERACTIVE GIRL

THE DIET INFORMATION provided in this book is not recommended as a long-term plan for any child. The Hyperactivity Test Diet is a short-term, four-week experiment to determine whether or not the foods and chemicals that, in our experience, have most often affected children's behavior present a problem for your child.

Many of the foods eliminated in this experiment are highly nutritious. Milk and dairy products provide many of the nutrients necessary for the health and well-being of children. They should not be permanently removed from any child's diet unless your physician confirms a severe cow's milk intolerance. During this experiment while milk and dairy products are eliminated, your child's diet should be supplemented with calcium. Although many foods contain some calcium, it is very difficult to obtain sufficient amounts from the diet alone.

Recommendations for supplementation are included with the diet plan.

Vitamin D supplementation is also necessary on the diet. Dairy-processed milk has vitamin D added to it. It teams up with the milk so that the calcium can be absorbed by the body. During the months of the year that skin is exposed to sunshine, your child's body manufactures vitamin D. During the other periods of the year, he or she should be given fish liver oil (the capsules don't taste fishy) or another source of vitamin D.

The fruits and vegetables eliminated during the experiment are all excellent sources of important nutrients and should not be eliminated permanently unless they are poorly tolerated by your child. Most children receive much of their required vitamin C from the fruits and juices restricted on this diet. For this reason, it is important that you give your child the fruits, vegetables and juices permitted on the plan.

Recipes are included for additive-free whole wheat bread and hamburger buns. In most areas you should be able to find an additive-free brand of whole wheat bread, rolls and pita bread. If you can't, your local baker will likely be agreeable to preparing a special order for you, especially if you are willing to take one to two dozen loaves of bread and a couple of dozen buns. You can be assured that the bread contains suitable ingredients if you provide them, and do ask that the pans, dividers and other surfaces that come in contact with the dough be oiled with an acceptable additive-free oil (see Appendix B). If you enjoy the mental and physical therapy of kneading bread, by all means make your own. Pita bread is not difficult to make, but it is time-consuming, and most of our children have tolerated the commercial varieties.

Most of the recipes in the Hyperactivity Test Diet don't require too much fuss, but you will spend some extra time cooking. Do prepare in advance, especially if you are a boil-in-the-bagger, can-opener, non-baking type of person. If you find the amount of cooking required overwhelming, try to enlist the help of a neighbor, friend or relative. Remember, this is only a four-week experiment.

If there is not a noticeable change in your little terror with the diet trial, either it is unlikely that diet is affecting his behavior, or it is possible that there are foods remaining in the diet that still cause problems. If this is the case, ask your doctor to refer you to a dietitian interested in the relationship between diet and hyperactivity, who will be able to help you evaluate the situation. Even if your child responds well to the diet trial, at the end of four weeks it will be time to start reintroducing foods to discover what makes your little time bomb tick and to add variety to the diet.

A bonus of the diet—if your entire family follows the prescribed menus—is that you may all feel better with more nutritious food that is higher in fiber and lower in sugar and additives than formerly. Once you have reintroduced low-fat milk and dairy products—if they are not a problem—and all or most fruits and vegetables, your diet will be first class.

DIET SPECIFICS

IF ALL THE FOODS AND CHEMICALS that children have reacted to were eliminated in this diet trial, the diet would be simple: it would consist of nothing. In this trial, only the items to which children have most often had behavioral reactions are eliminated. Families with youngsters who have many food allergies will be unlikely to find this trial useful. They should work with their physician and dietitian to come up with an individualized plan that will eliminate and then reintroduce possible food allergens. In addition to the foods eliminated in this diet, other common irritants, in our experience, are peanut butter, wheat, eggs and naturally occurring salicylates and benzoates.

To give you some hints about which intolerances your

child may suffer from, some of the foods and chemicals eliminated in the Hyperactivity Test Diet are discussed below.

Milk and Dairy Products

The most common food allergen for children is cow's milk. Based on our clinical findings, the following tends to be true of children with cow's milk intolerance:

• There is a family history of milk intolerance.
• Child had problems with cow's milk/formula during infancy.
• Child loves milk and drinks it excessively or hates it.
• Child has a runny nose, mucus, frequent respiratory and/or ear infections, bad breath, headaches.

Chocolate and Cola

The second most common food allergen for children is chocolate and cola. Families reported the following characteristics when their children were intolerant of chocolate and cola:

• The child craved and/or binged on these products and reacted to them by becoming jittery or having an upset stomach.
• Child had noticeable behavioral reactions to these items.

Sugar

Sugar is an inexpensive source of fuel and has been overrated as a cause of hyperactivity. Most children tolerate some sugar. Very few children react to lightly sugared products eaten in conjunction with other foods or at the end of a meal. Occasionally, it is the source of the sugar—cane or beets—that the allergic child reacts to, or the chemicals used in processing. There is no indication that honey is better than sugar; in fact, the sources of honey, such as clover and buckwheat, may cause reactions in allergic people. From our experience, some children who have been diagnosed as hypoglycemic have responded well to fructose as a sugar substitute.

The following tends to be true of children who have an intolerance for sugar:

• Members of the child's family have a high sugar intake.
• There is a family history of diabetes and/or hypoglycemia.
• There may also be a family history of alcoholism or a very low tolerance for alcohol.
• Child must eat often or is very crabby.
• Child has extreme sweet tooth—sneaks sugar from the sugar bowl, begs sweets from neighbors. Some even steal sweets from the corner store!

Artificial Colors and Flavors

It has been suggested that tartrazine (yellow dye #5) accounts for 85 percent of our artificial color intake. Tartrazine is found in a rainbow of colors, not just yellow. Since this dye often causes reactions other than hyperactivity (for example, asthma and hives), there has been pressure from the medical community to have it included on food and drug labels. Children have reactions to many other artificial colors and flavors, but it seems that tartrazine is the greatest offender. Most parents of hyperactive and even normal children report that their youngsters react to foods that are artificially colored, flavored and high in sugar. However, since these kinds of foods are often consumed on festive occasions, it is difficult to tell whether it is the food or the excitement of the party or holiday that causes the reaction. There are certain characteristics, though, that children who react to artificial color or flavor share. These are listed below:

• Child has a family background of intolerance, especially to tartrazine.
• Child has behavioral reactions to medications; for exam-

ple, becomes hyperactive after taking cough medication or antibiotics.
• Child has specific reactions to certain colored or flavored foods; for example, grape pop, cheese puffs, red gelatin.

Caffeine

Children's responses to caffeine-containing products can be a source of confusion for parents. Occasionally a child will calm down when given tea or coffee, but become shaky after having chocolate, cocoa or cola. The explanation for this could be that the child is allergic to elements other than the caffeine in the chocolate and cola family of food. It has been suggested that children who have adverse responses to the stimulant drugs used to control hyperactivity are also likely to have adverse responses to caffeine. Generally, children who become hyperactive after having caffeine:

• Respond negatively to stimulant drugs.
• Become jittery when given coffee or tea.
• Have parents who are intolerant of caffeine-containing products or are addicted to them.

Aspartame and Other Artificial Sweeteners

There is no scientific proof that aspartame (trade names are Equal and NutraSweet) given by itself causes hyperactivity. However, to my knowledge, research has not been done evaluating aspartame in conjunction with other products, such as the artificial colors and flavors that may be found in pop and gelatin desserts sweetened with it. Many parents have reported that their children become hyperactive, sleep poorly, have headaches and complain of stomachaches when they have foods or drinks containing aspartame. There would thus appear to be little merit in feeding this particular chemical to young children. The use of other artificial sweeteners is discouraged as well.

Monosodium Glutamate

Monosodium glutamate (MSG) is a flavor enhancer. In other words, it can zip up the taste of stale foods. It may be added to many processed foods: soups, meal mixes, frozen entrées, salad dressings, seasoning salts, sauces, processed meats and snack foods.

People who are intolerant of MSG are often intolerant of hydrolyzed vegetable protein (HVP) and hydrolyzed plant protein (HPP). Very sensitive people may also react to the high free glutamate levels in tomatoes, mushrooms and peas. Reactions to MSG have been dubbed Chinese Restaurant Syndrome, because MSG has been traditionally used in Chinese cuisine. Recently MSG has been linked with delayed onset asthma in some people. In our clinical experience, it has been a common behavioral irritant to hyperactive children. The following tends to be true of youngsters who react to MSG:

- Child has a family history of MSG intolerance.
- Child's parent suffers from Chinese Restaurant Syndrome.
- Child and parent have unexplainable gastrointestinal upsets and headaches.
- Child becomes bold, aggressive or cheeky after eating foods high in MSG.
- Child exhibits repetitive behaviors after eating foods containing MSG; for example, rocking, banging or making funny noises. We often observed this reaction in our clinical patients. One mother reported that her hyperactive son made Woody Woodpecker sounds for hours after eating at a fast food restaurant.

Benzoates

Benzoates include benzoic acid, sodium benzoate and benzoate of soda. They are preservatives, which under acidic conditions can prevent the growth of most micro-organisms. Some foods frequently containing preservative benzoates are pop, margarine, jam and pickles. They also occur naturally in most berries, prunes, tea and spices (cinnamon, cloves and anise). Children who appear to be intolerant of benzoates may:

• Dislike cinnamon and suntan screens and lotions containing PABA (paraminobenzoic acid).
• Be prone to hives, eczema or asthma.

We have also observed agitation, nausea, vomiting and cramping in these children.

BHT and BHA
Butylated hydroxytoluene (BHT) and butylated hydroxyanisole (BHA) are added to foods to preserve freshness and prevent rancidity. This means that you can open a box of cornflakes, forget it for six months, blow off the dust, eat them, and they'll still taste fresh. BHT and BHA are often added to breads, crackers, cereals, oil and fats, and high-fat snack foods. In our experience, BHT and BHA intolerance has not been nearly as common as intolerance to the items just discussed, but kids who are intolerant of these preservatives drive parents to distraction. One parent who had one of these little terrors said, "You know, he whined and hung on to my jean leg for so long that I finally grabbed the scissors, cut off the jean leg, gave it to him, and he continued to lug it around for hours, but at least he didn't bug me." Children who appear to be intolerant of these additives generally:

• Exhibit whiny, weepy behavior and are easily distracted for hours after they have eaten foods containing BHT and BHA. A good example is the happy morning riser who turns into a whiner after eating most prepared breakfast cereals.
• Come from a family who have recently emigrated from a country where the use of BHT and BHA is not permitted.

NON-FOOD FACTORS

IN ADDITION TO having food allergies, some children are intolerant of non-food items, such as scented products or substances found in the environment, for example, pollens or dust. Such children usually have parents with similar intolerances. Among the most common things they react to are: perfumes, soaps, detergents, toiletries, nail polish remover, ammonia, paint, paint thinner, markers, auto exhaust, cigarette smoke and strong cleansers.

CHAPTER FIVE

How To Chart Reactions

Discovering food sensitivities and isolating just what does what seems a very difficult, time-consuming activity, but the changes in our daughter certainly make it all very rewarding.
—MOTHER OF A FOUR-YEAR-OLD HYPERACTIVE GIRL

Keeping records may appear to be a chore. However, there are some definite advantages to doing so. All too quickly we can forget how bad things were before they got better. Also, if you chart the particular problems your youngster has in a diary like the one on page 31, you will see much more clearly, with time, the areas affected by diet. Ideally, you will keep daily records for a week prior to beginning the experiment and for the four weeks of the diet trial. Try to resist the temptation to compare days until the experiment is over.

Our studies show that the behavioral, sleep-related problems and physical symptoms included in the following lists can be alleviated by the diet trial. Choose the five most serious problems your child has from each list, then rate them daily as follows:

0 = Not at all, no sign of the problem or symptom
1 = Just a little, somewhat, not severe
2 = Severe, extreme, very exasperating

Total your scores daily; with time it is likely that the scores will decrease. However, it is unlikely that your child's scores will decrease immediately. In fact, allergists have reported an onslaught of symptoms when food allergens and caffeine are first removed from a patient's diet. Our observation has been that the first week is generally the worst. Our clinical experience with milk exclusion shows that it often takes ten to twelve days for the physical symptoms to subside, then an improvement in behavior has been observed. On the other hand, if a child is intolerant of food additives, stimulants and sugar, an improvement may be seen fairly quickly.

Behavioral Problems
• Excessive activity
• Disturbs other children
• Fails to finish things
• Short attention span
• Constantly fidgeting
• Inattentive, easily distracted
• Demands must be met immediately, easily frustrated
• Cries often and easily
• Unhappy, sulky
• Temper outbursts, explosive and unpredictable behavior
• Rapid mood swings
• Repetitive activity, words or sounds

If a short attention span is a major concern, note how long your child plays with a favorite toy or engages in a favorite activity on a daily basis. If there are other particularly annoying characteristics that you wish to monitor, add them to your list. Some examples parents have noted are: making "fish faces," stealing and hiding family possessions, chewing the bed and swearing.

Sleep-Related Problems
• Has trouble falling asleep
• Wakes up during the night

- Get up during the night (monitor number of times)
- Is very hot, damp during the night
- Is irritable, tired in the morning
- Is a bedwetter (note number of accidents)

Physical Symptoms
Physical symptoms that may be related to diet are numerous. In our experience, symptoms most frequently found to be altered by a diet trial are:

- Bad breath
- Stuffy, runny nose
- Headaches

Other reported and clinically observed physical symptoms include the following:

- Flushing
- Swelling of the hands, feet, face, tongue, lips
- Nosebleeds
- Vomiting and/or severe abdominal cramps
- Severe itching
- Eczema and other rashes
- Asthma
- Persistent breathing difficulties
- Repeated clearing of the throat, excessive mucus
- Darkness, puffiness, bags under the eyes
- Leg and foot cramps
- Bloated stomach or abdomen
- Excessively large bowel movements
- Very foul-smelling bowel movements
- Excessive gas
- Diarrhea
- Constipation
- Alternating diarrhea and constipation
- Itchiness, redness around genitals and/or anus

Many other symptoms have been reported, from glazed eyes to red ears. If you have noticed others that are frequent, add them to your list.

Keeping track of diet slipups and other such mishaps mentioned below could also help you solve the diet puzzle.

- Anyone who says that they never, ever have any diet slipups is immediately suspect. If your child eats something that is not on the diet plan, write it down. It could explain the flare-up of a certain symptom.
- Exposure to strong odors and possible reactions should be noted.
- A new puppy, a visit from grandma, a birthday party and other exciting events can very definitely affect behavior and sleep. If these incidents are noted, you will not confuse their effects with the effects of diet.
- Who more than hyperactive kids walks into walls, falls off windowsills, trips on the stairs and sticks their fingers into electrical sockets? If a mishap is serious enough to cause you more than momentary concern, record it.
- If medications must be given, they should be recorded in the daily diary. If they are colored or flavored, they could cause adverse reactions. If possible, drugs used to control hyperactivity should be tested before or after the diet trial. However, physicians frequently suggest doing diet and drug therapy at the same time. If you follow this course, you will still be able to monitor changes in physical symptoms and sleep patterns. But remember to use medications only on the advice of your physician, and ask that uncolored, unflavored medications be prescribed.

You can use the page that follows to monitor the changes in your child over the course of the diet trial. Photocopy the page thirty-five times so that you can keep daily records for a week before starting the diet trial and for the four weeks of the actual experiment.

THE FOOD EXPERIMENT DIARY

DATE _____   **DAY IN THE EXPERIMENT** _____

BEHAVIORAL PROBLEMS: SCORE   SCORE:

1. _____   _____   0 = Not at all

2. _____   _____   1 = Little

3. _____   _____   2 = Lots

4. _____   _____

5. _____   _____

SLEEP PROBLEMS

1. _____   _____

2. _____   _____

3. _____   _____

4. _____   _____

5. _____   _____

PHYSICAL PROBLEMS

1. _____   _____

2. _____   _____

3. _____   _____

4. _____   _____

5. _____   _____

   TOTAL DAILY SCORE   _____

DIET MISTAKES _____

_____

IMPORTANT SOCIAL EVENTS _____

_____

ACCIDENTS _____

_____

OTHER _____

_____

THE CHILD IN DAYCARE, PLAYSCHOOL OR SCHOOL

IT IS EXTREMELY FRUSTRATING to go to the work of carrying out all the steps of the diet trial to a tee at home only to find that they have been ignored away from home. Actually, if you describe the possible benefits of the plan to your child's caregivers, it shouldn't be difficult to enlist their help. It is unlikely that your child is a devil at home and an angel elsewhere. In all probability, he is a Dennis the Menace away from home, and his caregivers will be happy to help in any way they can. In addition to watching the diet, they may be willing to monitor behavior, because their work will be easier if your child is better behaved in the future. To ensure consistency, it is important to have the same person do the behavior rating each day.

If your child is in an extended daycare situation, you should go over the daycare menu with the cook and director and highlight the foods that your child can have. If you are permitted, it would be wise to take a look at the kitchen inventory. Frequently, for example, juices may be misrepresented. Strawberry juice may be apple juice with strawberry flavoring. Homemade soups may indeed have fresh vegetables, but they may be made with a soup base. It is unfair to expect the daycare center to purchase a number of special items for your child. You are much more likely to enlist their cooperation if you offer to provide the fill-in-the-gap items such as uncolored butter, acceptable bread, crackers and peanut butter.

In the diet trials we conducted, some of the parents of playschool and school-aged children provided all the snacks for the whole class if the groups were small. Another possibility is to go over the menus, noting dates and providing suitable substitute snacks for the days that the school's snacks are inappropriate.

It is important that caregivers record diet errors and

unusual events for you. Many cases of bizarre behavior have been reported after children with food intolerances have been exposed to spice-sniffing experiments, cleansers, perfumes, party foods, fingerpainting and foot painting. A sample record follows on the next page which you can photocopy and give to your child's caregiver to fill in.

THE FOOD EXPERIMENT DIARY FOR DAYCARE AND SCHOOLS

DATE _____ DAY IN THE EXPERIMENT _____

NAME OF CHILD _____

RECORDER'S NAME _____

BEHAVIORAL PROBLEMS:	SCORE	SCORE:
1. _____	_____	0 = Not at all
2. _____	_____	1 = Little
3. _____	_____	2 = Lots
4. _____	_____	
5. _____	_____	

   TOTAL SCORE   _____

DIET MISTAKES _____
_____

IMPORTANT SOCIAL EVENTS _____
_____

OTHER NOTES _____
_____
_____
_____

CHAPTER SIX

THE HYPERACTIVITY TEST DIET

My son had been on this diet for a week when we started to notice a difference in him. His behavior improved, his coldlike symptoms disappeared, and he slept better. As a result, he was able to concentrate better at school, was less frustrated, and his disposition improved.

—MOTHER OF A SIX-YEAR-OLD HYPERACTIVE BOY

I HAVE TRIED TO PROVIDE menus and recipes in this chapter and the next that use products that are readily available in small towns as well as large cities. Most of you, I hope, will have access to bakeries that will bake your breads and rolls with approved ingredients. If you are from a large center, you may find many additive-free products containing appropriate ingredients. Feel free to make substitutions, but do make sure that restricted items are not included on the labels. If a product is not labeled, as is the case for some dairy and deli items, avoid them for now. If you are lucky, you will find a sausage-maker who will prepare special bacon, ham, sausages and even hot dogs for you. However, do be very specific about permitted ingredients, especially spices.

In order to avoid milk and dairy products, it is important to be aware of ingredients which are milk-based. They are: milk solids, cheese, yogurt, cream, ice cream, lactose, caseinate or casein, lactalbumen, lactoglobulin, curds and whey. Even if there is an intolerance to the protein and milk sugar in other dairy products, butter is usually well tolerated and is used in this plan because it can be purchased without additives.

Usually, if sugar is not well tolerated, maple syrup, molasses, honey, the natural sugar in full-strength juice and other natural sweeteners will also cause problems. Generally, the solution is to use sugar modestly. Fruits and their juices contain moderate to high amounts of natural sugar. Moderate use of fruit and dilution of juice (one part water to one part juice) are advised. If a special, high sugar treat is part of a meal, give it to your child at the end of the meal, when he or she has a full, not an empty stomach. The sugar content in almost all regular recipes can be reduced by at least 50 percent. Recipes in this book usually have no more than 1 tsp (5 mL) sugar per muffin or cookie. Fruit desserts have a higher content of natural sugar.

The second part of this chapter contains detailed menus for a two-week period, which include notes that tell you how to plan ahead for the next day. The two-week cycle will be repeated to provide a four-week trial. You needn't worry about the diet being too repetitive, as recipes for varying the second cycle are included. Just before the detailed daily menus, you will find a summary of the menus, or menus at a glance, so that you can quickly scan the meal plan for the days ahead. The actual recipes follow in the next chapter.

The one important thing to note here is that the meals for the two-week menu have been carefully planned to provide all the needed nutrients (except calcium and vitamin D) for the average four-to six-year-old. Nutrient analysis of the menus was done with the NUTS Nutrition Assessment System Version 3.3. By increasing or decreasing portion sizes, this plan can be adjusted to be nutritionally adequate for any age and either sex. (See more about these adaptations for different ages in Appendix A.)

Prediet Game Plan

BEFORE BEGINNING THE DIET, you will need to get rid of foods that are not allowed on the diet. If your family loves snacks, you probably have bowls of mints, crunchy salted nuts and tempting fruit around the house. The refrigerator and freezer are probably loaded with tempting goodies, and the cupboards are full of gourmet delights. The only reasonable plan is to eat them up or lock them up prior to starting the diet. Many of the families that we have counseled have chosen to wait two to three weeks to begin the diet. There are several advantages of doing this:

• Food is not wasted because you have time to eat it up.
• You make room in your refrigerator and freezer for diet items.
• If you want to rate your child's behavior prior to the diet and get used to keeping a diary, this is a good time to do so.
• The delay will give you time to remove environmental allergens, such as scented items.
• Much of the baking for the diet can be done in advance so that you will not be overwhelmed with the extra baking and different cooking methods used during the experiment.
• In many cases, the delay has allowed parents to trade, sell or give away items that are unsuitable for the diet.
• Giving yourself extra time also allows you to store items that you can't use or don't want to get rid of.

Supplementation

THE DAILY NUTRIENT INTAKE on the Hyperactivity Test Diet will be adequate except for calcium and vitamin D. There are many supplements on the market which can fill your child's needs. Basically, the four-to six-year-old requires 600 mg of calcium per day. This diet plan averages 335 mg of calcium per day. Therefore a supplement of 250 to 300 mg of usable or elemental calcium per day should be sufficient. The daily requirement of vitamin D for this age group is 200 IU of vitamin D (5 ug cholecalciferol). Since the diet provides an average of 65 IU of vitamin D, your child will require a supplement of 125 to 150 IU per day. This is a small supplement, but it will be essential during the months when your child's skin is not frequently exposed to direct sunlight. The amount of supplementation can be easily adjusted for other age groups; adaptation information is provided in Appendix A.

There are several calcium supplements on the market containing varying amounts of elemental calcium. Some of these supplements also contain vitamin D. Discuss your needs with your pharmacist, who is the expert in this area. Remember to ask for calcium supplements that are free of artificial colors, flavors and preservatives and that also contain a limited amount of sugar.

How To Use The Appendices

YOU MAY FIND IT HELPFUL to consult the Appendices before beginning the diet.

Appendix A provides you with some suggestions for adapting the menus for other members of the family.

Appendix B contains a list of food products which are suitable for use on this diet. Undoubtedly, there are many appropriate foods that are not listed here that you may add as you find them.

Appendix C provides you with a limited list of toiletries, cleaning supplies and art supplies that most children with allergies will tolerate. It also lists environmental allergens, such as cigarette smoke and gas and oil. If your child's problems are mostly caused by environmental allergens, you should consult your allergist for advice as this is not my area of expertise.

You are now ready to begin the Hyperactivity Test Diet. Good luck and away you go!

MENUS AT A GLANCE

DAY 1	DAY 2	DAY 3	DAY 4
BREAKFAST	BREAKFAST	BREAKFAST	BREAKFAST
Peanut Butter	Honey-Maple	Hamwich	Egg
Toasties	Walnut	Pineapple Juice	Whole Wheat
Lemonade	Oatmeal		Toast
	Lemonade		Pineapple Juice
SNACK	SNACK	SNACK	SNACK
Gorp	Fruit Kabob	Digestive	Gorp
		Cookies	
LUNCH	LUNCH	LUNCH	LUNCH
Super Soup	Pick-Up-Sticks	Beanpot Baked	Carrot-Pear
Rye Crackers	Lunch	Lentils	Soup
Banana	Peanut Cookie	Whole Wheat	Bran Muffin
Lemonade	Lemonade	Bread	Pineapple Juice
		Mouse Salad	
		Pineapple Juice	
SNACK	SNACK	SNACK	SNACK
Frozen Peas	Peach Slurpee	Tropicalsicle	Melon Cubes
DINNER	DINNER	DINNER	DINNER
Chinese	Almost Ham	Fat Fish Fingers	Oven-Baked
Chicken Wings	Homemade	Oven French	Chicken
Brown Rice	Mustard	Fries	Funny Sort of
Stir-Fried	Sweet Potato	Rhubarb	Scalloped
Vegetables	Casserole	Ketchup	Potatoes
Soya Sauce	Raw Broccoli	Coleslaw	Green Beans
Instant Fruit	Blueberry Muffin	Oatmeal Cookie	Pickled Beets
Sherbet	Lemonade	Pineapple Juice	Oatmeal Cookie
Lemonade			Pineapple Juice
BEDTIME	BEDTIME	BEDTIME	BEDTIME
Digestive	Peanuts	Whole Wheat	Digestive
Cookies	Lemonade	Bread	Cookies
Lemonade		Peanut Butter	Pineapple Juice
		Pineapple Juice	
SUPPLEMENTS	SUPPLEMENTS	SUPPLEMENTS	SUPPLEMENTS
Calcium	Calcium	Calcium	Calcium
Vitamin D	Vitamin D	Vitamin D	Vitamin D

DAY 5	**DAY 6**	**DAY 7**	**DAY 8**
BREAKFAST	BREAKFAST	BREAKFAST	BREAKFAST
Instant Energy Cereal	Pineapple Granola	Campers' Pancakes	Bran Muffin Peanut Butter
Limeade	Limeade	Honey-Maple Syrup	Honey Jungle Juice
		Jungle Juice	
SNACK	SNACK	SNACK	SNACK
Banana	Ants on a Log	Peanutsicle	Banana Bumps
LUNCH	LUNCH	LUNCH	LUNCH
Chicken Pita Pocket	Dippy Lunch Blueberry Muffin	Tuna on a Bun Dill Pickle	Chicken Noodle Soup
Green Pepper Ring Bracelet	Limeade	Pear Jungle Juice	Rice Crackers Raw Carrot
Ladybug Cookie			Candlestick
Lemonade			Salad
			Jungle Juice
SNACK	SNACK	SNACK	SNACK
Frozen Cherries or Blueberries	Pear Slurpee	Gorp	Cherries
DINNER	DINNER	DINNER	DINNER
Tasty Hamburger with Trimmings	Linguine with White Clam Sauce	Marinated Flank Steak	Almost Sausage Pattie
Oven French Fries	Tossed Salad Haupt Dressing	Foil-Wrapped Potato and Onion	Homemade Mustard
Rhubarb Ketchup	Breadstick Worms	Mixed Vegetables	Hobo Vegetables
Raw Carrot	Banana Sherbet	Banana Cake	Jellied Fruit
Peanut Cookie	Limeade	Jungle Juice	Lemonade
Limeade			
BEDTIME	BEDTIME	BEDTIME	BEDTIME
Digestive Cookie	Healthy Banana Bread	Digestive Cookie	Breadstick Worm
Raspberry Fizz	Lemonade	Jungle Juice	Lemonade
SUPPLEMENTS	SUPPLEMENTS	SUPPLEMENTS	SUPPLEMENTS
Calcium	Calcium	Calcium	Calcium
Vitamin D	Vitamin D	Vitamin D	Vitamin D

DAY 9	**DAY 10**	**DAY 11**	**DAY 12**
BREAKFAST	BREAKFAST	BREAKFAST	BREAKFAST
Island Cereal	Scrambled Egg	Pineapple	Peanut Butter
Green Giant	Whole Wheat	Granola	Toasties
Drink	Toast	Pink Drink	Pink Drink
	Green Giant		
	Drink		
SNACK	SNACK	SNACK	SNACK
Gorp	Healthy Banana	Whole Wheat	Fruit Kabob
	Bread	Bread	
	Green Giant	Peanut Butter	
	Drink	Pink Drink	
LUNCH	LUNCH	LUNCH	LUNCH
Peanut Butter	Meatloaf	Little Red Hen	Winter Barley
Toasties	Sandwich	Salad	Soup
Turnip Sticks	Digestive	Whole Wheat	Rye Crackers
Canteloupe	Cookies	Bread	Raw Carrot
Chunks	Carrot-	Oatmeal Cookie	Ladybug Cookie
Green Giant	Pineapple	Pink Drink	Pear
Drink	Cocktail		Pink Drink
SNACK	SNACK	SNACK	SNACK
Apricotsicle	Peach Slurpee	Bananasicle	Apricotsicle

DINNER	DINNER	DINNER	DINNER
Power-Packed Meatloaf	Pineapple-Baked Chicken	Fishburger	Spaghetti and Marvelous
Rhubarb Ketchup	Brown Rice	Bean Salad	Meat Sauce
Potato Chips	Mixed Vegetables	Peach or Nectarine	Tossed Greens
Kids' Guacamole	Peanut Cookie	Pink Drink	Haupt Salad Dressing
and Raw Veggies	Green Giant Drink		Banana Cake
Pineapple Sherbet			Pink Drink
Green Giant Drink			

BEDTIME	BEDTIME	BEDTIME	BEDTIME
Healthy Banana Bread	Ants on a Log	Digestive Cookies	Digestive Cookies
Green Giant Drink	Green Giant Drink	Pink Drink	Lemon Fizz

SUPPLEMENTS	SUPPLEMENTS	SUPPLEMENTS	SUPPLEMENTS
Calcium	Calcium	Calcium	Calcium
Vitamin D	Vitamin D	Vitamin D	Vitamin D

Day 13

BREAKFAST
Bran Muffin
Peanut Butter
Honey
Fruit Drink

SNACK
Pineapple
 Granola
Lemonade

LUNCH
Shrimp Salad
Potato Salad
Lettuce
Raw Carrot
Rye Cracker
Banana
Fruit Drink

BEDTIME
Fruit Slice
 Sandwich

DINNER
Sweet and Sour
 Turkey
Brown Rice
Soya Sauce
Lettuce Wedge
Boiled Dressing
Oatmeal Cookie
Fruit Drink

BEDTIME
Potato-Skin
 Crisps
Sparkling Water

SUPPLEMENTS
Calcium
Vitamin D

Day 14

BREAKFAST
Whole Wheat
 French Toast
Honey-Maple
 Syrup
Fruit Drink

SNACK
Digestive
 Cookies
Fruit Drink

LUNCH
Yuppie Grazer
 Lunch
Blueberry Muffin
Parsley Surprise

BEDTIME
Snow Cone

DINNER
Veal Stew
Hot Casserole
 Bread
Ladybug
 Cookies
Fruit Drink

BEDTIME
Toasted
 Almonds
Fruit Drink

SUPPLEMENTS
Calcium
Vitamin D

MENUS

DAY 1 MENU

BREAKFAST   Peanut Butter Toasties:
Spread 2 slices of whole wheat toast with 1 tbsp (15 mL) peanut butter. Make a sandwich and cut into 5 strips.
½ cup (125 mL) lemonade
Don't forget to add 6 cans of water to 1 can concentrate.

SNACK   5 Tbsp (75 mL) Gorp:
Mix together ¼ cup (50 mL) puffed wheat, 1 tbsp (15 mL) sunflower seeds, 1 tbsp (15 mL) flaked coconut and 1 tbsp (15 mL) currants.

LUNCH   1 cup (250 mL) Super Soup*
2 Ryvita rye crackers
1 small banana
½ cup (125 mL) lemonade

SNACK   ¼ cup (50 mL) frozen peas in a small cup

DINNER   4 pieces (2 wings) Chinese Chicken Wings*
Make plenty of leftovers for lunch tomorrow.
½ cup (125 mL) Brown Rice*
¼ cup (50 mL) Stir-Fried Carrots, Peppers and Onions*
1 tsp (5 mL) soya sauce (optional)
½ cup (125 mL) Instant Fruit Sherbet*
Try pears packed in their own juice.
½ cup (125 mL) lemonade

BEDTIME   2 Digestive Cookies*
½ cup (125 mL) lemonade

SUPPLEMENTS   250-300 mg calcium and 125-150 IU vitamin D

NOTES FOR TOMORROW
• Put a can of peaches in their own juice in the freezer for tomorrow's afternoon snack slurpee.
• Marinate Almost Ham* for tomorrow's supper. If possible, begin this dish early today to provide enough marinating time.
* Recipes provided

DAY 2 MENU

BREAKFAST   Honey-Maple Walnut Oatmeal:
Add 2 tbsp (25 mL) Honey-Maple Syrup* and 1
tbsp (15 mL) walnuts to ½ cup (125 mL)
Oatmeal*
½ cup (125 mL) lemonade

SNACK   1 Fruit Kabob:
Assemble 2 1-inch slices banana, 2 1-inch cubes
melon, 2 ½-inch slices kiwi fruit. Have child string
fruit on wooden skewer.

LUNCH   Pick-Up-Sticks Lunch*
1 Peanut Cookie*
½ cup (125 mL) lemonade

SNACK   ½ cup (125 mL) Peach Slurpee*:
Blend frozen peaches and juice in food processor
or blender and serve with a short straw.

DINNER   2 oz (60 g) Almost Ham*
Save some ham for tomorrow's breakfast.
1 tsp (5 mL) Homemade Mustard* (optional)
½ cup (125 mL) Sweet Potato Casserole*
2 raw broccoli florets (or trees), 1½oz (45 g)
1 Blueberry Muffin*
1 tsp (5 mL) butter
½ cup (125 mL) lemonade

BEDTIME   3 tbsp (45 mL) peanuts
½ cup (125 mL) lemonade

SUPPLEMENTS   250-300 mg calcium and 125-150 IU vitamin D

NOTES FOR TOMORROW
• Make Tropicalsicles* for tomorrow's afternoon snack.
• Coleslaw* for tomorrow's dinner will be better if you make it a day
ahead.
* Recipes provided

DAY 3 MENU

BREAKFAST   Hamwich:
Place 1 oz (30 g) of Almost Ham* between 2
slices of whole wheat bread buttered with 1 tsp (5
mL) of butter.
½ cup (125 mL) pineapple juice
Don't forget to dilute juice 1:1 with water.

SNACK   2 Digestive Cookies*

LUNCH   ¾ cup (175 mL) Beanpot Baked Lentils*
1 slice whole wheat bread
½ tsp (2 mL) butter
1 Mouse Salad*
½ cup (125 mL) pineapple juice

SNACK   1 Tropicalsicle*

DINNER   2 oz (60 g) Fat Fish Fingers*
lemon wedge (optional)
½ cup (125 mL) Oven French Fries*
1 tbsp (15 mL) Rhubarb Ketchup*
½ cup (125 mL) Coleslaw*
1 Oatmeal Cookie*
½ cup (125 mL) pineapple juice

BEDTIME   1 slice whole wheat bread
2 tsp (10 mL) peanut butter
½ cup (125 mL) pineapple juice

SUPPLEMENTS   250-300 mg calcium and 125-150 IU vitamin D

NOTES FOR TOMORROW
Surprise—no work!
* Recipes provided

DAY 4 MENU

BREAKFAST   1 egg, poached, boiled or scrambled (with water)
1 slice whole wheat toast
½ tsp (2 mL) butter
½ cup (125 mL) pineapple juice

SNACK   Gorp:
Mix together 2 tbsp (25 mL) peanuts, 2 halves
dried apricots, slivered, 1 tbsp (15 mL) sunflower
seeds and 2 tbsp (25 mL) puffed rice.

LUNCH   ¾ cup (175 mL) Carrot-Pear Soup*
1 Bran Muffin*
1 tsp (5 mL) butter
½ cup (125 mL) pineapple juice

SNACK   ½ cup (125 mL) melon, cubed
Try using honeydew melon.

DINNER   3 oz (90 g) Oven-Baked Chicken*
Without the bones, this should equal
approximately 2 oz. Make enough for lunch
tomorrow.
½ cup (125 g) Funny Sort of Scalloped Potatoes*
¼ cup (50 mL) green beans
¼ cup (50 mL) Pickled Beets*
1 Oatmeal Cookie*
½ cup (125 mL) pineapple juice

BEDTIME   2 Digestive Cookies*
½ cup (125 mL) pineapple juice

SUPPLEMENTS 250-300 mg calcium and 125-150 IU vitamin D

NOTES FOR TOMORROW
Surprise again—no work!
* Recipes provided

DAY 5 MENU

BREAKFAST   Instant Energy Cereal:
Add 2 tsp (10 mL) peanut butter, 1 tbsp (15 mL)
peanuts, chopped, and 1 tsp (5 mL) honey to ½
cup (125 mL) Oatmeal*.
½ cup (125 mL) limeade
Don't forget to add 6 cans of water to 1 can of
concentrate.

SNACK   1 small banana

LUNCH   Chicken Pita Pocket:
Fill ½ of a small Pita Bread* with ¼ cup (50 mL)
diced chicken, 2 tbsp (25 mL) chopped celery,
1 tbsp (15 mL) Old-Fashioned Boiled Dressing*
and 1 tbsp (15 mL) Zucchini Relish*.
1 Green Pepper Ring Bracelet:
Child can wear the slice of green pepper while
eating pita pocket, then eat the bracelet.
1 Ladybug Cookie*
½ cup (125 mL) lemonade

SNACK   ¼ cup (50 mL) frozen blueberries
Frozen sweet cherries are a good substitute.

DINNER   1 Tasty Hamburger:
1 Tasty Burger* pattie
1 whole wheat bun
1 tsp (5 mL) Rhubarb Ketchup* (optional)
1 tsp (5 mL) Zucchini Relish* (optional)
1 tsp (5 mL) Homemade Mustard* (optional)
1 lettuce leaf
1 slice onion (optional)
½ cup (125 mL) Oven French Fries*
1 tbsp (15 mL) Rhubarb Ketchup*
1 small carrot, cut into strips or left whole
1 Peanut Cookie*
½ cup (125 mL) limeade

BEDTIME   1 Digestive Cookie*
1 Raspberry Fizz:
In a glass, mix ½ cup (125 mL) sparkling water

with 1 tbsp (15 mL) frozen raspberry juice concentrate. Add ice and a short straw.

SUPPLEMENTS 250-300 mg calcium and 125-150 IU vitamin D

NOTES FOR TOMORROW
• Put a can of pears in their own juice in the freezer for tomorrow's afternoon Pear Slurpee* snack.
• Make Banana Sherbet*.
* Recipes provided

DAY 6 MENU

BREAKFAST   ⅓ cup (75 mL) Pineapple Granola*
                ½ cup (125 mL) limeade

SNACK   Ants on a Log:
                    Spread ½ stalk of celery with 2 tsp (10 mL)
                    peanut butter and decorate with 5 currant ants.

LUNCH   Dippy Lunch*
                1 Blueberry Muffin*
                1 tsp (5 mL) butter
                ½ cup (125 mL) limeade

SNACK   ½ cup (125 mL) Pear Slurpee*

DINNER   Linguine with White Clam Sauce:
                    Cover ½ cup (125 mL) cooked linguine with ⅓
                    cup (75 mL) White Clam Sauce*.
                ½ cup (125 mL) tossed salad
                    Use lettuce and any other raw vegetables you
                    have left over.
                Haupt Salad Dressing*
                2 Breadstick Worms*
                    Use leftovers from lunch.
                ½ cup (125 mL) Banana Sherbet*
                ½ cup (125 mL) limeade

BEDTIME   1 slice Healthy Banana Bread*
                ½ cup (125 mL) lemonade

SUPPLEMENTS 250-300 mg calcium and 125-150 IU vitamin D

NOTES FOR TOMORROW
• Make Peanutsicles* for tomorrow morning.
• Make the Beef Marinade* and pour it into a 13 × 9-inch (33 × 23-cm) pan. Place a flank steak in the marinade, turn it, and cover with foil or plastic wrap. Turn steak a couple of times before cooking it tomorrow evening.
* Recipes provided

DAY 7 MENU

BREAKFAST   4 Campers' Pancakes*
3 tbsp (45 mL) Honey-Maple Syrup*
½ cup (125 mL) Jungle Juice*

SNACK   1 Peanutsicle*

LUNCH   Tuna on a Bun:
Spread ¼ of the Tuna Salad* recipe on 1 whole wheat hamburger bun. Or toast the bun, spread it with salad and heat under the broiler.
½ dill pickle
1 small pear
½ cup (125 mL) Jungle Juice*

SNACK   Gorp:
Mix together 2 tbsp (25 mL) almonds, 2 tbsp (25 mL) sunflower seeds, 1 tsp (5 mL) carob chips and 2 tbsp (25 mL) puffed rice.

DINNER   2 oz (60 g) barbecued or broiled Marinated Flank Steak:
Barbecue or broil the steak after marinating it in Beef Marinade* overnight. Try slicing the cooked meat on the diagonal. You will find it very tender.
1 Foil-Wrapped Potato and Onion*
Mixed Vegetables:
Mix together and microwave or boil 2 tbsp (30 mL) mushrooms, 2 tbsp (30 mL) peas and 2 tbsp (30 mL) cauliflower.
2 oz (60 g) Banana Cake*
½ cup (125 mL) Jungle Juice*

BEDTIME   2 Digestive Cookies*
½ cup (125 mL) Jungle Juice*

SUPPLEMENTS   250-300 mg calcium and 125-150 IU vitamin D

NOTES FOR TOMORROW
Surprise! No work.
* Recipes provided

DAY 8 MENU

BREAKFAST 1 Bran Muffin*
1 tbsp (15 mL) peanut butter
1 tsp (5 mL) honey
½ cup (125 mL) Jungle Juice*

SNACK Banana Bumps:
Spread 1 Ryvita rye cracker with 2 tsp (10 mL)
peanut butter. Top it with 2 slices of banana each
½inch (1 cm) thick.

LUNCH 1 cup (250 mL) Chicken Noodle Soup*
1 or 2 rice crackers
1 tsp (5 mL) butter
1 whole small carrot
1 Candlestick Salad*
½ cup (125 mL) Jungle Juice*

SNACK ¼ cup (50 mL) fresh or frozen cherries

DINNER 2 oz (60 g) Almost Sausage Pattie*
2 tsp (10 mL) Homemade Mustard* (optional)
1 packet Hobo Vegetables*
½ cup (125 mL) Jellied Fruit*
½ cup (125 mL) lemonade

BEDTIME 1 Breadstick Worm*
½ cup (125 mL) lemonade

SUPPLEMENTS 250-300 mg calcium and 125-150 IU vitamin D

NOTES FOR TOMORROW
• Make Apricotsicles* for tomorrow's afternoon snack. Pour ¼ cup
(50 mL) of unsweetened apricot nectar into each popsicle cup. If
you make enough for Day 12, too, you will not need to make them
again.
• For tomorrow night's dinner make Pineapple Sherbet using the
Instant Fruit Sherbet* recipe.
* Recipes provided

DAY 9 MENU

BREAKFAST   Island Cereal:
On top of ½ cup (125 mL) Oatmeal* sprinkle ½ banana, sliced, 1 tbsp (15 mL) coconut and 1 tsp (5 mL) brown sugar.
½ cup (125 mL) Green Giant Drink*

SNACK   ⅓ cup (75 mL) Gorp:
Mix together 2 tbsp (25 mL) puffed rice, 2 tbsp (25 mL) sunflower seeds, 2 tsp (10 mL) currants and 1 tsp (5 mL) carob chips.

LUNCH   Peanut Butter Toasties:
Spread 1 tbsp (15 mL) of peanut butter on 2 slices of whole wheat toast. Cut into 5 strips.
½ cup (125 mL) turnip sticks
1 cup (250 mL) canteloupe chunks
½ cup (125 mL) Green Giant Drink*

SNACK   1 Apricotsicle*

DINNER   2 oz (60 g) Power-Packed Meatloaf*
Save some for tomorrow's lunch.
1 tbsp (15 mL) Rhubarb Ketchup* (optional)
1 oz (30 g) potato chips
¼ recipe Kids' Guacamole Dip*
4 oz (125 g) of a variety of raw vegetable dippers
Pick from asparagus, broccoli, cabbage, carrots, cauliflower, celery, cucumber, green or yellow beans, jicama, mushrooms, peppers, radishes, snow peas, turnip, zucchini—just use whatever you have on hand.
⅓ cup (75 mL) Pineapple Sherbet
Use the Instant Fruit Sherbet* recipe.
½ cup (125 mL) Green Giant Drink*

BEDTIME   1 slice Healthy Banana Bread*
½ cup (125 mL) Green Giant Drink*

SUPPLEMENTS   250-300 mg calcium and 125-150 IU vitamin D

NOTES FOR TOMORROW
• Freeze a can of peaches that were canned in their own juice for tomorrow afternoon's Peach Slurpee* snack.
* Recipes provided

DAY 10 MENU

BREAKFAST 1 egg scrambled with water and 1 tsp (5 mL) butter
1 slice whole wheat toast
½ tsp (2 mL) butter
½ cup (125 mL) Green Giant Drink*

SNACK 1 slice Healthy Banana Bread*
½ cup (125 mL) Green Giant Drink*

LUNCH Meatloaf Sandwich
On 2 slices whole wheat bread spread 1 tsp (5
mL) butter, 1 tsp (5 mL) Old-Fashioned Boiled
Dressing*, and 1 tsp (5 mL) Homemade
Mustard*. Mustard is optional. Between the bread
place
1 leaf of lettuce and 1½ oz (45 g) Meatloaf*.
2 Digestive Cookies*
¾ cup (175 mL) Carrot-Pineapple Cocktail*

SNACK ½ cup (125 mL) Peach Slurpee*

DINNER 2 oz (60 g) Pineapple-Baked Chicken*
Save some of the chicken for tomorrow's lunch.
Weight is the measure of boned chicken.
2 tbsp (30 mL) sauce from Pineapple-Baked
Chicken*
½ cup (125 mL) Brown Rice*
¼ cup (60 mL) cooked mixed vegetables
Try cauliflower, celery and green beans in equal
amounts.
½ tsp (2 mL) butter
1 Peanut Cookie*
½ cup (125 mL) Green Giant Drink*

BEDTIME Ants on a Log
Spread ½ stalk of celery with 2 tsp (10 mL) peanut
butter and decorated with 5 currant "ants."
½ cup (125 mL) Green Giant Drink*

SUPPLEMENTS 250-300 mg calcium and 125-150 IU vitamin D

NOTES FOR TOMORROW
• Make a Bananasicle. Cut a banana in half, insert a popsicle stick
and freeze.
* Recipes provided

DAY 11 MENU

BREAKFAST   ⅓ cup (75 mL) Pineapple Granola*
             ½ cup (125 mL) Pink Drink*

SNACK   1 slice whole wheat bread
             2 tsp (10 mL) peanut butter
             ½ cup (125 mL) Pink Drink*

LUNCH   Little Red Hen Salad*
             1 slice whole wheat bread
             ½ cup (2 mL) butter
             1 Oatmeal Cookie*
             ½ cup (125 mL) Pink Drink*

SNACK   1 Bananasicle*

DINNER   Fishburger:
                 In 1 whole wheat hamburger bun place 2 tsp (10
                 mL) Old-Fashioned Boiled Dressing* (optional), a
                 lettuce leaf, and 1 Salmon Burger*.
             lemon wedge (optional)
             ½ cup (125 mL) Bean Salad*
             1 small peach or nectarine
             ½ cup (125 mL) Pink Drink*

BEDTIME   2 Digestive Cookies*
             ½ cup (125 mL) Pink Drink*

SUPPLEMENTS 250-300 mg calcium and 125-150 IU vitamin D

NOTES FOR TOMORROW
• Make Apricotsicles for tomorrow's afternoon snack if you do not
  have leftovers from Day 9.
* Recipes provided

DAY 12 MENU

BREAKFAST   Peanut Butter Toasties:
                Spread 2 slices of whole wheat toast with 1 tbsp
                (15 mL) peanut butter. Cut into 5 strips.
              ½ cup (125 mL) Pink Drink*

SNACK   Fruit Kabob:
                On a skewer string ½ small banana cut in 3
                chunks and 4 frozen cherries (slightly thawed).

LUNCH   1 cup (250 mL) Winter Barley Soup*
              2 Ryvita rye crackers
              1 small carrot left whole
              1 Ladybug Cookie*
              1 small pear
              ½ cup (125 mL) Pink Drink*

SNACK   1 Apricotsicle*

DINNER   Spaghetti and Marvelous Meat Sauce:
                Pour ½ cup (125 mL) Marvelous Meat Sauce* over
                ½ cup (125 mL) cooked spaghetti.
              ½ cup (125 mL) tossed greens with Haupt Salad
                Dressing*
              2 oz (60 g) Banana Cake*
              ½ cup (125 mL) Pink Drink*

BEDTIME   2 Digestive Cookies*
              1 Lemon Fizz:
                Mix ½ cup (125 mL) sparkling water with 1 tbsp
                (15 mL) lemonade concentrate.

SUPPLEMENTS   250-300 mg calcium and 125-150 IU vitamin D

NOTES FOR TOMORROW
None!
* Recipes provided

DAY 13 MENU

BREAKFAST   1 Bran Muffin*
1 tbsp (15 mL) peanut butter
1 tsp (5 mL) honey
½ cup (125 mL) Fruit Drink*

SNACK   ¼ cup (50 mL) Pineapple Granola*
½ cup (125 mL) lemonade

LUNCH   ¼ recipe Shrimp Salad*
½ cup (125 mL) Potato Salad*
   Bake 6 medium potatoes. Carefully cut potatoes
   in half and carefully remove the potatoes from
   their skins. Skins will be used for bedtime
   snack.
1 lettuce leaf
1 small carrot, cut into strips
1 Ryvita rye cracker
1 small banana
½ cup Fruit Drink*

SNACK   Fruit Slice Sandwich
   Cut 2 pear slices, each ¼inch (½cm) thick.
   Spread 1 tbsp (15 mL) peanut butter between the
   2 to make sandwich.

DINNER   ¾ cup (175 mL) Sweet and Sour Turkey*
   Simmered chicken can be used as a substitute for
   the turkey.
½ cup (125 mL) Brown Rice*
2 tsp (10 mL) soya sauce (optional)
1 small lettuce wedge
2 tsp (10 mL) Old-Fashioned Boiled Dressing*
1 Oatmeal Cookie*
½ cup (125 mL) Fruit Drink*

BEDTIME   4 Potato-Skin Crisps*
   Use the skin of 1 potato.
½ cup (125 mL) sparkling water

SUPPLEMENTS 250-300 mg calcium and 125-150 IU vitamin D

NOTES FOR TOMORROW
None again!
* Recipes provided

DAY 14 MENU

BREAKFAST   1 slice Whole Wheat French Toast*
                   2 tbsp (30 mL) Honey-Maple Syrup*
                   1 tsp (5 mL) butter
                   ½ cup (125 mL) Fruit Drink*

SNACK   2 Digestive Cookies*
                   ½ cup (125 mL) Fruit Drink*

LUNCH   Yuppie Grazer Lunch:
                       Surround a bowl of ¼ recipe of Dandy Bean Dip*
                       with ½ Pita Bread* cut into scoopers and 4 oz
                       (125 g) of a variety of vegetable dippers. See Day
                       9 for vegetable suggestions.
                   1 Blueberry Muffin*
                   1 tsp (5 mL) butter
                   ⅓ cup (75 mL) Parsley Surprise*

SNACK   1 Snow Cone*

DINNER   1 cup (250 mL) Veal Stew*
                   1 slice Hot Casserole Bread*
                   1 tsp (5 mL) butter
                   2 Ladybug Cookies*
                   ½ cup (125 mL) Fruit Drink*

BEDTIME   2 tbsp (25 mL) toasted almonds
                       Toast in oven at 135°C (275°F) until golden.
                   ½ cup (125 mL) Fruit Drink*

SUPPLEMENTS 250-300 mg calcium and 125-150 IU vitamin D
* Recipes provided

CHAPTER SEVEN

Recipes, Recipes, Recipes

Our whole family followed the diet, and as a bonus our other son stopped having the ear infections he was very prone to.

—MOTHER OF A FIVE-YEAR-OLD HYPERACTIVE BOY

THE RECIPES IN THIS CHAPTER are divided into three sections. The first section contains recipes that can be prepared in advance. The second section includes recipes for the two-week cycles. In the third section, you will find alternate recipes, which allow you to add variety to the second two-week cycle. Within the sections, the recipes are organized by category.

Make-Ahead Recipes

SOUPS

Super Soup (Day 1)
Combine in a large pot:

2 lb	soup bones		1 kg
14 cups	water		3.5 L
8 oz	pot barley		250 g
8 oz	soy beans		250 g
2 tsp	salt		10 mL
2	bay leaves		2

Simmer for 3-4 hours. Remove the bones. Separate the meat from the bones, chop the meat and add to the soup broth along with 8 cups (2 L) of chopped vegetables. The following are only suggestions. Feel free to substitute.

1 lb	cabbage, chopped	500 g
1 lb	carrots, chopped	500 g
1	medium onion, diced	1
12 oz	outer celery stalks and leaves, diced	375 g
8 oz	frozen peas	250 g
2 oz	parsley, chopped	60 g
2	cloves of garlic, finely chopped	2
½ lb	lean ground beef	250 g

Bring to a boil. Stir well and simmer for 45 minutes to an hour. Add water to bring yield to 20 cups (5 L). Add salt and pepper to taste.

Note: The addition of basil, oregano, thyme to taste and cooked broken up spaghetti will turn this soup into Minestrone.

Yield: 20 cups (5 L)

Chicken Noodle Soup (Day 8)

4 cups	chicken broth (made from chicken parts, 1 onion, bay leaf, celery leaves and 6 cups (1.5 L) water)	1 L
½ cup	chopped celery	125 mL
1½ cups	cooked noodles	375 mL
1½ cups	cooked diced chicken	375 mL

Heat broth and add celery. Simmer for 5 minutes. Add the noodles and chicken. Add salt and pepper to taste. Add enough water to bring the yield to 6 cups (1.5 L).

Note: Chicken backs make good inexpensive soup. To save a pot and extra cooking time, add 2 oz (60 g) of dry noodles directly to the soup. Let the noodles cook 10-15 minutes, again adding enough water to bring the final yield to 6 cup (1.5 L). To give soup a little extra zing, add chopped fresh parsely and chopped green onion tops.

Yield: 6 cups (1.5 L)

Winter Barley Soup (Day 12)

Adapted from a recipe in the *Good Housekeeping Cookbook*

2.5 lb	beef or lamb stew meat, chopped small	1.2 kg
2 tbsp	uncolored butter	25 mL
6 cups	boiling water	1.5 L
½ cup	pot barley	125 mL
2	medium onions, sliced	2
2 tbsp	parsley, chopped	25 mL
1 tsp	salt	5 mL
¼ tsp	pepper	1 mL
1	bay leaf	1
1½ cups	chopped celery	375 mL
1½ cups	diced carrots	375 mL
½ tsp	thyme	2 mL

In a Dutch oven, brown meat in butter over medium high heat. Add 6 cups (1.5 L) of hot water, barley, 1 sliced onion, parsley, salt, pepper and bay leaf. Heat to boiling. Reduce heat to low, and simmer covered for 1½ hours.

Stir in the remaining sliced onion and the rest of the ingredients, and cook for 30 minutes or until the meat is fork tender. Discard the bay leaf. Add salt if you must and pepper to taste.

Yield: Approximately 11 cups (2.75 L)

BAKING

Digestive Cookies (Days 1, 3, 4, 5, 7, 10, 11, 12, 14)

Adapted from a recipe in the La Leche League cookbook, *Whole Foods for the Whole Family*

1½ cups	untreated whole wheat flour	375 mL
½ cup	rolled oats	125 mL
¼ cup	wheat germ	50 mL
¼ cup	sesame seeds	50 mL
¼ tsp	baking soda	1 mL
¼ tsp	salt	1 mL

3 tbsp	pure honey	45 mL
¼ cup	uncolored butter	50 mL
¼ cup	preservative-free oil	50 mL
⅓ cup	cold water	75 mL
1 tsp	pure vanilla extract	5 mL

Combine the dry ingredients in a large bowl. Cut in butter to make coarse, even crumbs. Combine water, honey, vanilla and oil; drizzle over flour mixture. Blend until dough can be packed into a ball.

Roll dough into a 2-inch (5-cm) diameter roll. Wrap it in waxed paper and freeze until firm.

Unwrap dough and slice it into ⅛ -inch (3-mm) thick cookies. Bake on greased cookie sheets (using an oil that has no preservatives) at 325°F (160°C) for 20-25 minutes. They should brown only slightly. Store in an airtight container.

Yield: 30 cookies weighing approximately ⅓ oz (10 g) each

Peanut Cookies (Days 2, 5, 10)

1 cup	untreated whole wheat flour	250 mL
½ cup	rolled oats	125 mL
⅓ cup	wheat germ	75 mL
¼ tsp	salt	1 mL
¼ tsp	baking soda	1 mL
1½ cups	recommended infant cereal	375 mL
¼ cup	chopped preservative-free peanuts	50 mL
¼ cup	uncolored butter	50 mL
¼ cup	pure peanut butter	50 mL
½ cup	pure honey	125 mL
1	egg, beaten	1
1 tsp	pure vanilla extract	5 mL

In a bowl, combine the first 7 ingredients. In another bowl, cream the butter, peanut butter and honey together until the mixture is smooth. Add and beat in the egg and vanilla. Then mix in dry ingredients. Shape the dough into a roll approximately 2 inches (5 cm) in diameter. Wrap well in waxed paper and chill or freeze until firm.

Slice the dough into ⅛ -inch (3-mm) slices. Place on ungreased cookie sheets and bake in a preheated 350°F (180°C) oven for 10-14 minutes or until crisp.

Yield: 42 cookies weighing approximately ½ oz (15 g) each

Oatmeal Cookies (Days 3, 4, 11, 13)
Use recipe for Peanut Cookies with the following changes:

1. Omit peanuts and peanut butter.
2. Add ¼ cup (50 mL) of preservative-free oil.

Ladybug Cookies (Days 5, 12, 14)

1½ cups	untreated whole wheat flour	375 mL
½ cup	packed light brown sugar	125 mL
½	uncolored butter	125 mL
2	eggs	2
¼ tsp	salt	1 mL
½ tsp	pure vanilla extract	2 mL
¼ tsp	baking soda	1 mL
2 tbsp	carob powder	25 mL
	carob chips or dried currants	

Measure the first 7 ingredients and place in a large bowl. Beat with a mixer until well mixed. Spoon 3 tbsp (45 mL) of the dough into a small bowl. Add carob powder to the small bowl and work it in. Wrap both balls of dough in waxed paper and refrigerate for at least 1 hour. Preheat oven to 350°F (180°C).

Cut the light dough into 36 pieces. Shape each piece with a 1 tsp (5 mL) measuring spoon. Drop onto a cookie sheet greased with preservative-free oil, 1 inch (2.5 cm) apart.

With a blunt knife draw a deep line lengthwise down the center of each cookie. Press two carob chips or currants on each side of the line. Shape carob dough into 36 pea-sized balls. Flatten a ball on one end of each cookie to resemble the head of a ladybug. Bake 12-15 minutes until light brown.

Yield: 36 cookies

Blueberry Muffins (Days 2, 6, 14)

¾ cup	untreated white flour	175 mL
1 cup	untreated whole wheat flour	250 mL
4 tsp	baking powder	20 mL
¼ tsp	salt	1 mL
¼ cup	white sugar	50 mL
1 cup	recommended infant cereal	250 mL
1	egg	1
1 cup	unsweetened pineapple juice	250 mL
¼ cup	preservative-free oil	50 mL
1 cup	frozen unsweetened blueberries	250 mL

In a large bowl, mix together the first 6 ingredients. In another bowl, beat the egg, juice and oil until well blended. Add this mixture to the dry ingredients and mix just until blended. Fold in the blueberries.

Divide the batter evenly into 12 muffin tins greased with preservative-free oil. Sprinkle each muffin with a pinch (½ mL) of white sugar. Bake at 400°F (200°C) for 25 minutes.

Yield: 12 muffins weighing approximately 2 oz (60 grams) each

Bran Muffins (Days 4, 8, 13)

1 cup	untreated whole wheat flour	250 mL
1 tsp	baking soda	5 mL
1 tsp	baking powder	1 mL
¼ tsp	salt	250 mL
1 cup	recommended infant cereal	375 mL
1½ cups	bran	425 mL
1¾ cups	water	50 mL
¼ cup	molasses	1
1	egg, beaten	125 mL
½ cup	dried currants	

In a large bowl, combine the first 6 ingredients until evenly blended. Add the beaten egg, molasses and water. Stir until the dry ingredients are well mixed. Fold in the currants.

Grease 17 muffin cups with preservative-free oil or use white paper liners. Place an equal amount of batter in each cup. Bake for 20 minutes at 375°F (190°C)

Yield: 17 muffins weighing approximately 2 oz (55 g) each

Healthy Banana Bread (Days 6, 9, 10)

1 cup	preservative-free oil	250 mL
1 cup	lightly packed brown sugar	250 mL
6	eggs, beaten	6
1 tsp	salt	5 mL
2 tbsp	pure lemon juice	25 mL
2 cups	water	500 mL
2 tsp	pure vanilla extract	10 mL
2 cups	ripe bananas, mashed or puréed (about 8)	500 mL
4 cups	untreated whole wheat flour	1 L
⅔ cup	wheat germ	150 mL
2 tsp	baking soda	10 mL

In a large bowl, cream the sugar and oil. Add the eggs, bananas and salt. In another large bowl, mix together the flour, wheat germ and soda. In a large measuring cup, combine the water, lemon juice and vanilla. To the banana mixture add alternately the dry ingredients and the mixture of water, lemon and vanilla.

Pour the batter into 4 bread pans well oiled with preservative-free oil. Bake at 350°F (180°C) for 35-45 minutes. Let cool on a rack before removing them from the pans.

Note: This recipe can be halved quite easily.

Yield: 4 loaves, each 20 slices

Banana Cake (Days 7, 12)

3	eggs	3
½ cup	pure honey	125 mL
3	bananas, peeled and sliced	3
1 tsp	pure vanilla extract	5 mL
½ cup	preservative-free oil	125 mL
½ cup	chopped walnuts	125 mL
2 cups	untreated whole wheat flour	500 mL
1 tbsp	baking powder	15 mL

Preheat the oven to 325°F (160°C). Oil a 13 × 9 × 2-inch (33 × 23 × 5-cm) pan with preservative-free oil. In a blender, combine the eggs, honey, bananas, vanilla and oil. Blend until smooth. Add the walnuts and turn the blender on and off quickly just to mix.

In a large bowl, stir together the flour and baking powder. Pour the blender mixture over the flour and mix well. Pour the batter into the baking pan. Bake for approximately 30 minutes or until an uncolored toothpick inserted in the middle of the cake comes out clean. Let cool on a wire rack.

Yield: Total recipe yields 35 oz (1.1 kg) or 24 pieces weighing 1½ oz (45 g) each

If you cannot purchase preservative-free, milk-free bread, here are a few recipes for either you or your baker to make.

Freezer Whole Wheat Bread

6 cups	untreated whole wheat flour	1.5 L
7 cups	untreated white flour (approximately)	1.75 L
4 pkg	active dry yeast	4 pkg
3 tbsp	white sugar	45 mL
2 tsp	salt	10 mL
4 cups	water	1 L
⅓ cup	molasses	75 mL
¼ cup	uncolored butter	50 mL
1	egg white	1

This recipe can be made up to a month before it is needed.

In a large bowl, combine the whole wheat flour with 6 cups (1.5 L) of the white flour. In another bowl, combine the yeast, sugar, salt and 2 cups (500 mL) of the flour mixture. In a 2 qt (2 L) saucepan heat the water, molasses and butter over a low heat until the butter is almost melted.

With the mixer at low speed, gradually beat the liquid into the yeast, sugar and flour mixture until just blended. Increase speed to medium and beat for 2 more minutes, occasionally scraping the bowl with a rubber spatula. Beat in 2½ cups (625 mL) of the mixed flours to make a thick batter. Continue beating for 2 minutes, occasionally scraping the bowl. With a wooden spoon, stir in the remaining flour mixture to make a soft dough.

Turn dough onto a lightly floured surface and knead, gradually working in more white flour, about 1 cup (250 mL). Knead dough until smooth and elastic, approximately 10 minutes. Shape dough into a ball. Cover and let it rest for 15 minutes. Meanwhile, grease 4 bread pans with a preservative-free oil.

Cut dough into 4 pieces. Shape each piece into an oval and place in a bread pan. Cover with plastic wrap and freeze until firm. Remove from pans and wrap in foil or place in individual freezer bags. Seal, label and freeze. (See Note.)

About 5 hours before serving, remove as many bread loaves as needed from the freezer. Unwrap and place in bread pans greased with a preservative-free oil. Let stand at room temperature, loosely covered in waxed paper until completely thawed. This takes about 2 hours.

In a cup, beat the egg white slightly with a fork. Brush dough lightly with the egg white. Then let rise in a warm place 80-85°F (26-28°C), away from drafts, until it has more than doubled in size. This takes about 2 hours.

Preheat oven to 375°F (190°C). Bake bread for 35 minutes or until the loaf sounds hollow when lightly tapped. Remove from pans, and cool on a wire rack.

Note: If you wish to bake the bread without freezing, cover the freshly made dough with a towel and let rise in a warm place until it has more than doubled in size, about 1 hour. Bake as directed.

Yield: 4 loaves, each 16 slices

Hamburger Buns

4 cups	untreated whole wheat flour	1 L
4 cups	untreated white flour	1 L
2 pkg	active dry yeast	2 pkg
2 cups	warm water	500 mL
¾ cup	preservative-free oil	175 mL
¼ cup	white sugar	50 mL
1 tsp	salt	5 mL
3	eggs	3

In a large mixing bowl, combine 2 cups (500 mL) of whole wheat flour, 2 cups (500 mL) white flour and the yeast. Combine warm water, oil, sugar and salt. Add this to the dry mixture in the bowl. Add the eggs and beat at low speed, scraping the sides of the bowl constantly. Beat for 3 minutes at high speed. By hand, stir in enough of the remaining flour to make a soft dough. Turn out on a lightly floured surface and knead until smooth. Place in a bowl greased with preservative-free oil, turning once to grease all surfaces. Cover and let rise until it has doubled in size. This takes about 1 hour.

Punch down the dough and divide into 3 portions. Cover and let rest for 5 minutes. Divide each portion of dough into 8 pieces. Shape each piece into a round ball and press flat. Place on baking sheet greased with preservative-free oil, and press to 3½ -inch (9-cm) circles. Let rise until double in size, about 30 minutes.

Bake in a 375°F (190°C) oven for 10 minutes. Remove from sheets and let cool on a wire rack.

Yield: 24 buns

Pita Bread

1 cup	lukewarm water	250 mL
1 pkg	active dry yeast	1 pkg
1 tbsp	white sugar	15 mL
½ tsp	salt	2 mL
1 tsp	preservative-free oil	5 mL
1 cup	untreated whole wheat flour	250 mL
1¾ cups	untreated white flour	425 mL

In a large bowl, mix water, yeast and sugar. Let stand until bubbly. Stir in oil and salt. Gradually stir in 2 cups (500 mL) of the flour or enough to make a stiff dough. Turn dough out on a lightly floured surface, and knead for about 10 minutes or until smooth and elastic. Place the dough in a bowl lightly greased with preservative-free oil. Turn the dough once to grease the top. Cover and let rise in a warm place for about an hour or until it has doubled in size.

Turn out on a lightly floured surface. Cut into 8 equal pieces. Roll each into a ball and then flatten with fingers to a 4-inch (10-cm) round. Let rest for 5-10 minutes. With a rolling pin, roll each ball out to make a 6-inch (15-cm) round. Place on heavily floured waxed paper or a board. Cover with waxed paper and a light towel. Let rise in a warm, draft-free place for 30 minutes or until the rounds look smooth and slightly raised.

Meanwhile, place a heavy baking sheet in the middle of the lowest oven rack. There should be 2.5 inches (7 cm) between the oven rack and the oven walls. Preheat oven to 500°F (250°C). After about 20 minutes of preheating, carefully transfer the rounds with a pancake turner or a metal spatula. Being careful not to tear dough, place them floured-side down onto the heated pan. Bake for 4-5 minutes or until the loaves balloon up and are lightly browned.

Remove the loaves from the oven and place on waxed paper. Cover with more waxed paper and a towel. Loaves will soften with their own steam as they cool. Cool, and then press down to flatten each loaf. Store in plastic bags. To serve, cut in half crosswise, and pull open to make 2 pockets.

Yield: 8 pita breads

BREAKFAST DISHES

Pineapple Granola (Days 6, 11, 13)

6 cups	quick-cooking rolled oats	1.5 L
1 cup	unsweetened pineapple juice	250 mL
½ cup	wheat germ	125 mL
2 tsp	pure vanilla extract	10 mL
½ cup	chopped dates	125 mL
½ cup	shredded unsweetened coconut	125 mL
½ cup	sunflower seeds	125 mL

Mix the oats thoroughly with the pineapple juice. Bake on 1 or 2 cookie sheets in a 325°F (160°C) oven until dry and golden brown. Stir frequently. Combine the remaining ingredients, add to the oats, and mix thoroughly. Store in an airtight container.

Yield: One recipe yields 6½ cups (1.6 L) weighing 26 oz (800 g)

Campers' Pancakes (Day 7)
Mix:

2 cups	untreated whole wheat flour	500 mL
2 tbsp	soy milk powder (optional)	25 mL
2 tbsp	baking powder	25 mL
¼ tsp	salt	1 mL
½ cup	wheat germ	125 mL

For each cup of mix add:

1 cup	water	250 mL
1	egg, beaten	1

Oil a grill well with preservative-free oil. Cook pancakes using a scant 2 tbsp (25 mL) of batter for each pancake.

Yield: 1 cup (250 mL) of mix makes 18 small pancakes of approximately 1 oz (28 g) each.

ADDED TOUCHES

Honey-Maple Syrup (Days 2, 7, 14)
Combine:

¼ cup	dark pure honey	50 mL
¼ cup	pure maple syrup	50 mL
4 tsp	untreated white flour	20 mL
1 cup	cold water	250 mL

Combine all ingredients in a saucepan and stir well until blended. Heat until mixture simmers and thickens.

Yield: a scant 1½ cups (350 mL)

Homemade Mustard (Days 2, 5, 8, 13)

1 tbsp	untreated white flour	15 mL
¼ cup	white sugar	50 mL
¼ tsp	salt	1 mL
2 tbsp	dry mustard	25 mL
⅓ cup	water	75 mL
¼ cup	white vinegar	50 mL

In a pot, blend vinegar, water and dry ingredients until smooth. Cook over low heat, stirring constantly, until smooth and thick. Pour into a glass jar and refrigerate. A small amount of turmeric can be added for coloring, but it will change the flavor of the mustard.

Yield: ⅔ cup (150 mL)

Rhubarb Ketchup (Days 3, 5, 9)

4 cups	chopped rhubarb	1 L
½ cup	water	125 mL
¼ cup	chopped onions	50 mL
1¾ cups	brown sugar	425 mL

¼ cup	white vinegar	50 mL
½ tsp	salt	2 mL
¾ tsp	cinnamon	3 mL

Combine the rhubarb, water, onion, sugar and vinegar in a saucepan. Bring to a boil slowly, stirring frequently. Simmer, still stirring, until thick. Add salt and cinnamon, and simmer for 5 more minutes. Cool, and purée the mixture in a blender. Reheat and simmer, stirring frequently, until desired consistency. Refrigerate.

Yield: Varies depending on how long it is cooked and how much water has evaporated.

Pickled Beets (Day 4)

1 lb	small beets (approximately 13)	500 g
	boiling salted water	
4	whole allspice	4
½ cup	white vinegar	125 mL
4 tsp	white sugar	20 mL
½ tsp	salt	2 mL

Scrub beets well. Trim the stems about ½ inch (2.5 cm) from the top of each beet. In a medium-sized saucepan, cook, covered in boiling salted water, until the skins slip off easily. This takes about 35-40 minutes. Drain, and when cool enough to handle, slip off the skins. Slice and transfer to a clean jar.

Meanwhile, crush allspice slightly. In a small pan, heat the vinegar, salt, sugar and allspice until boiling. Pour over the beet slices, and stir to coat evenly. Let stand until cool. Cover and refrigerate for at least 2 hours before serving.

Yield: 2 cups (500 mL)

Zucchini Relish (Days 5, 11)

¾ lb	zucchini, chopped	375 g
1	large onion, chopped	1
½ cup	white vinegar	125 mL
2 tsp	salt	10 mL
¼ tsp	baking soda	1 mL

Scrub the zucchini well; cut off both ends and chop into fine pieces. (A food processor does an excellent job with zucchini and onion.) Place all the ingredients in a pot and bring to a boil. Simmer until most of the liquid has evaporated. Refrigerate.

Yield: Approximately 1 lb (500 g)

Old-Fashioned Boiled Dressing (Days 5, 10, 11, 13)

1	egg	1
2 tbsp	white sugar	25 mL
2 tbsp	untreated white flour	25 mL
⅓ cup	white vinegar	75 mL
1 tsp	salt	5 mL
1 cup	water	250 mL

Whisk together all ingredients in a heavy saucepan or in the top of a double boiler. Cook, stirring constantly, until thickened. Cool and store in a glass container in the refrigerator.

Yield: 1¾ cups (425 mL)

Homemade Butter

(Only if you cannot buy uncolored butter)

2 cups	whipping cream	500 mL
¼ cup	ice cold water	50 mL
	salt to taste	

Whip cream in a food processor or blender until thick. Add water and continue mixing until the cream separates. Turn into a strainer and hold under cold running water, kneading the mixture to remove as much of the white, milky liquid as possible. Pat dry with white paper towels. Mix in salt if desired. Mold into desired shape and refrigerate for at least 30 minutes before serving.

OTHER HYPERACTIVITY TEST DIET RECIPES

SOUPS AND SALADS

Carrot-Pear Soup (Day 4)

4	carrots, peeled and cut in chunks	4
1	onion, peeled and finely cut	1

1	pear, peeled and cut in pieces	1
4 cups	chicken stock	1 L
¼ tsp	thyme	1 mL
	Salt to taste	

Place all ingredients except salt in a saucepan. Simmer for 10 minutes or until the carrots are tender. Whip in the blender until smooth. Add salt to taste.

Yield: Approximately 6 cups (1.5 L)

Pick-Up-Sticks Lunch (Day 2)

2	Chinese Chicken* pieces	2
½	celery stalk, cut in strips	½
1	small carrot, pared and cut in strips	1
1	slice whole wheat toast	1
½ tsp	spread with uncolored butter	2.5 mL

Have the child drop all of the above items on a plate. Either a parent or another child determines the order in which different foods will be consumed (without disturbing the surrounding foods). When the child does disturb or move another food, he or she stops eating and establishes the order in which food will be eaten by his or her meal companion. The child does not resume eating until his or her partner moves a non-specified food. This is lots of fun for two people, but it is time-consuming for more than two.

Yield: 1 serving

Mouse Salad (Day 3)

Place an unsweetened, canned pear half, cut side down, on a leaf of lettuce. Cut two slits on the sides of the small end of the pear, and insert two carrot coins for ears. Press in two currants for eyes, a sunflower seed for a mouth and a carrot stick for a tail.

Yield: 1 serving

Coleslaw (Day 3)

| 3 lb | cabbage (1 medium) | 1.5 kg |
| ¼ cup | white sugar | 50 mL |

½ cup	white vinegar	125 mL
3 tbsp	preservative-free oil	45 mL
1 tsp	salt	5 mL
1 tsp	celery seed	5 mL

Shred cabbage and sprinkle with sugar. In a saucepan, simmer vinegar, oil, salt and celery seed for 10 minutes. Pour over the cabbage. Cover and refrigerate for 6-8 hours.

Yield: 10 cups (2.5 L)

Dippy Lunch (Day 6)

⅓ cup	Chick Dip*	75 mL
2	Whole Wheat Breadstick Worms*	2
1	broccoli floret	1
¼	celery stalk, cut in strips	¼
1	small carrot, pared and cut in strips	1
⅛	green pepper, cut in strips	⅛
1	cauliflower floret	1

Put Chick Dip in a small bowl in the center of a plate. Surround the bowl with Breadstick Worms and the vegetables. Dip each item in the dip and eat.

Yield: 1 serving

Tuna Salad (Day 7)

1	can (7 oz/198 g) flaked tuna	1
½ cup	chopped green pepper	125 mL
¼ cup	chopped pimiento	50 mL
1 tbsp	lemon juice	15 mL
¼ cup	Old-Fashioned Boiled Dressing*	50 mL

Toss all ingredients together, and use salad as topping for Tuna Buns.*

Yield: 4 servings

Candlestick Salad (Day 8)

On a lettuce leaf place a drained, unsweetened pineapple slice. Insert ¼ of a banana for a candle. On the top of the banana candle press in a carrot-stick flame.

Yield: 1 serving

Haupt Salad Dressing (Days 6, 12, 13)

¼ cup	water	50 mL
¼ cup	preservative-free oil	50 mL
¼ cup	white vinegar	50 mL
½ tsp	salt	2 mL
½ tsp	white sugar	2 mL

Combine all ingredients and shake well.

Little Red Hen Salad (Day 11)
A Louise Lambert-Lagacé adaptation

½ cup	shredded carrot	125 mL
2 tbsp	finely chopped green pepper	25 mL
1 tbsp	Old-Fashioned Boiled Dressing*	15 mL

Toss together and form into a nest on a leaf of lettuce placed on a plate. Fill with:

| 1½ oz | cooked chicken, cut in chunks | 45 g |

Bean Salad (Day 11)

¼ cup	white sugar	50 mL
½ cup	preservative-free oil	125 mL
½ cup	white vinegar	125 mL
½ tsp	salt	2 mL
1 can	cut green beans, drained	1 can
1 can	cut wax beans, drained	1 can
1 can	red kidney beans, drained	1 can
1 can	garbanzo beans (chickpeas), drained	1 can
½ cup	finely chopped onion	125 mL

Mix the first 4 ingredients well. Toss with the vegetables and refrigerate.
   Yield: 10-12 servings

Potato Salad (Day 13)

| ½ cup | Old-fashioned Boiled Dressing* | 125 mL |
| 1 tbsp | white vinegar | 15 mL |

½ tsp	salt	2 mL
1 tsp	Homemade Mustard*	5 mL
¼ tsp	celery seed	1 mL
	dash of pepper	
6	potatoes, baked and diced	6
¼ cup	chopped green onion	50 mL
¼ cup	chopped parsley	50 mL

Mix the dressing with the next 5 ingredients. Carefully remove the skins from the potatoes (see recipe for Potato-Skin Crisps*), and dice the potato. Add remaining ingredients and mix well.

Yield: 4-6 servings

Shrimp Salad (Day 13)

1 can	shrimp, drained	1 can
1 cup	sliced celery	250 mL
¼ cup	chopped walnuts	50 mL
2 tsp	finely chopped onion	10 mL
3 tbsp	Old-Fashioned Boiled Dressing*	45 mL
3 tbsp	Haupt Salad Dressing*	45 mL

Combine all ingredients and mix well.

Yield: 4 small servings

MAIN COURSE DISHES

Chinese Chicken Wings (Days 1, 2)

10	chicken wings	10
¼ cup	white sugar	50 mL
¼ cup	pure soya sauce	50 mL
1 tsp	preservative-free oil	5 mL
1 tsp	garlic powder (or 1 large clove, pressed)	5 mL

Cut the wings at the joints so that each wing is in 3 pieces. Save wing tips for making stock. Place the remaining wing pieces in a bowl with the rest of the ingredients. Refrigerate for at least 30 minutes or, better still, overnight. Stir occasionally to keep wings covered with sauce.

Preheat the oven to 350°F (180°C). Grease a baking pan with preservative-free oil. Arrange the wings in a single layer in the pan, pouring any extra liquid on top. Bake for 45 minutes, turning after 20 minutes. Serve hot or cold.

Yield: 5 servings of 2 wings each (Recipe is approximately 40 percent bone.)

Almost Ham (Days 2, 3)
For each 2 lb (kg) of fresh pork roast mix together:

2 tsp	salt	10 mL
¼ tsp	pepper	1 mL
¼ tsp	crushed bay leaf	1 mL
¼ tsp	allspice	1 mL
1	clove garlic, pressed	1

Rub this mixture well into meat. Refrigerate for 2 days, turning twice a day. Dry before browning. Brown pork in 1 tbsp (15 mL) of preservative-free oil. Remove meat and sauté in the oil:

1	carrot, sliced
1	onion, sliced
1	small bunch parsley, chopped
½	bay leaf
1	clove garlic, finely chopped

Put sautéed vegetables into a pot. Add meat and a cup of stock or leftover vegetable water, and cook in a 350°F (170°C) oven until done. 3 lb (1.5 kg) cooks in approximately 2 hours.

Fat Fish Fingers (Day 3)

1 lb	firm white fish fillets (cod, sole, etc.)	500 g
½ cup	wheat germ	125 mL
¼ cup	sesame seeds	50 mL
¼ tsp	salt	1 mL
2	small eggs (or 1 large)	2
2 tbsp	preservative-free oil	25 mL

Grease a baking sheet with preservative-free oil. Preheat the oven to 350°F (180°C). Cut fish into 1 × 4-inch (2.5 × 10-cm) fingers. Mix wheat germ, sesame seeds and salt in a bowl. In another bowl, whisk eggs and oil. Roll fish in wheat germ mixture, soak in egg mixture, and then roll again in the wheat germ. Place on a baking pan and bake in oven for approximately 15 minutes.

Yield: 10 fingers weighing 2 oz (60 g) each

Oven-Baked Chicken (Days 4, 5)

1	large broiler chicken, cut up	1
¼ cup	uncolored butter	50 mL
¼ cup	untreated whole wheat flour	50 mL
½ tsp	salt	2 mL
¼ tsp	pepper	1 mL

Preheat the oven to 425°F (220°C). Melt the butter in a baking pan. Mix flour, salt and pepper in a plastic bag, and shake chicken pieces 2-3 at a time in this mixture. Put the coated chicken pieces in the pan, skin-side-down. Bake for 30 minutes. Turn and bake for 15 minutes longer or until skin is brown and crisp.

Yield: 4 servings

Tasty Burgers (Day 5)

1½ lb	lean ground beef	750 g
¾ cup	wheat germ	175 mL
½ cup	chopped onion	125 mL
1	egg	1
½ tsp	salt	2 mL
¼ tsp	pepper	1 mL

Combine all ingredients, mixing well. Shape into 10 patties of equal size. Broil 3-4 minutes on each side.

Yield: 10 patties, each 3 oz (90 g) raw weight 2 oz (60 g) cooked weight

White Clam Sauce (Day 6)

2 cans	minced clams, 5 oz (142 g) each	2 cans
3 tbsp	preservative-free oil	45 mL
1	clove garlic, minced	1
½ cup	chopped parsley	125 mL

| ¾ tsp | basil | 3 mL |
| ¼ tsp | salt | 1 mL |

Drain the clams and set aside their juice. In a medium saucepan over medium heat, cook garlic in hot oil until tender. Stir in the clam juice and remaining ingredients except the clams. Cook for 10 minutes, stirring occasionally. Add the clams. Cook until heated through.

Yield: Approximately 2 cups (500 mL) of sauce

Beef Marinade for Flank Steak (Day 7)

¼ cup	preservative-free oil	50 mL
2 tbsp	lemon juice	25 mL
½ tsp	salt	2 mL
½ tsp	oregano	2 mL
¼ tsp	pepper	1 mL
1	clove garlic, finely minced or pressed	1

Combine all ingredients and mix well. Use to marinate 1-2 lb (.5-1 kg) flank steak. Marinate for 24 hours, turning meat several times. Barbecue or broil the meat and slice on the diagonal.

Almost Sausage Patties (Day 8)

1 lb	ground pork	500 g
¼ tsp	coriander seeds, crushed	1 mL
½	bay leaf, crushed	½
½ tsp	salt	2 mL
½ tsp	pepper	2 mL
4 tsp	pure lemon juice	20 mL

Mix all ingredients well, and leave in the refrigerator for at least 6 hours. The patties may be cooked immediately, but the flavors blend better after standing. Shape into 6 patties and fry or broil until nicely browned and cooked all the way through.

Yield: 6 patties, each 3 oz (90 g) raw weight, 2 oz (60 g) cooked weight

Power-Packed Meatloaf (Days 9, 10)

| 1½ lb | lean ground beef | 750 g |
| 6 oz | beef liver, puréed in blender | 190 g |

2	eggs	2
2 cups	recommended infant cereal	500 mL
½ cup	wheat germ	125 mL
½ cup	chopped onion	125 mL
1 tsp	salt	5 mL
¼ tsp	pepper	1 mL
½ tsp	sage	2 mL
½ tsp	dry mustard	2 mL
⅓ cup	Rhubarb Ketchup*	75 mL

Preheat the oven to 325°F (160°C). Combine all ingredients and pack into a loaf pan. Bake for 90 minutes.

Yield: 2½ -lb (1.2 kg) loaf

Pineapple-Baked Chicken (Day 10)

2 lb	chicken parts (breasts are excellent)	1 kg
1 cup	unsweetened pineapple juice	250 mL
1 tsp	salt	5 mL
1 tsp	rosemary, crushed	5 mL
½ tsp	paprika	2 mL
¼ tsp	pepper	1 mL
2 tbsp	untreated white flour	25 mL

Preheat oven to 375°F (190°C). In a roasting pan, place chicken skin-side-up. Pour in the pineapple juice.

In a cup, combine salt, rosemary, paprika and pepper. Sprinkle over the chicken. Bake for 50-60 minutes or until fork tender, basting with pan juices occasionally.

Remove chicken to a warm platter and spoon fat from the pan juices. In a cup, blend flour and ¼ cup (50 mL) water until smooth. Gradually stir this mixture into the hot juices. Cook the sauce until slightly thickened. Serve with the chicken.

Yield: Varies with chicken parts used and size of serving desired

Salmon Burgers (Day 11)

| 2 | cans (7.5 oz/235 g) salmon (not packed in oil) | 2 |

½ cup	fine soft milk-free bread crumbs	125 mL
¼ cup	finely chopped onion	50 mL
2	eggs, slightly beaten	2
¼ cup	Zucchini Relish*	50 mL
1 tsp	lemon juice	5 mL
	Salt and pepper to taste	
	Dry, fine milk-free bread crumbs for coating	
2 tbsp	uncolored butter	25 mL

Drain salmon, and blend well with remaining ingredients except butter. Shape into 4 patties of equal size. Melt butter in a frying pan, and cook patties for about 4 minutes on each side, or until nicely browned.

Yield: 4 patties

Marvelous Meat Sauce (Day 12)

1 cup	canned mushrooms, drained	250 mL
1 cup	chopped onions	250 mL
1 cup	chopped celery	250 mL
2	cloves garlic, finely chopped or pressed	2
2 tbsp	preservative-free oil	25 mL
1 lb	lean ground beef	500 g
3 cups	canned or fresh pumpkin pulp	750 mL
1 cup	water	250 mL
1 tbsp	honey	15 mL
1 tsp	salt	5 mL
2 tbsp	white vinegar	25 mL
½ tsp	oregano	2 mL
½ tsp	basil	2 mL
½ tsp	thyme	2 mL
¼ tsp	pepper	1 mL
1 tsp	paprika	5 mL

Sauté the first 4 items in preservative-free oil. Set aside. In a large saucepan, brown the beef, and drain off any fat. Then add the rest of the ingredients to the beef. Add enough additional water to bring the mixture to the consistency of tomato sauce. The amount will depend on the thickness of the pumpkin pulp, but it will probably need about ⅔ -1½ cups (375 mL) of water. Simmer for approximately 30 minutes.

Yield: Varies depending on pulp, 4-6 servings

Sweet and Sour Turkey (Day 13)

14 oz	can peaches in their own juice	398 mL
1	medium onion, thinly sliced	1
1 cup	sliced celery	250 mL
½ cup	green pepper cut in strips	125 mL
3 tbsp	preservative-free oil	45 mL
¼ cup	pure soya sauce	50 mL
¼ cup	white vinegar	50 mL
2 tbsp	brown sugar	25 mL
2 tbsp	untreated white flour	25 mL
2 cups	cubed cooked turkey (pork or chicken)	500 mL

Drain peaches, reserving the juice. Set juice and peaches aside. In a large skillet, sauté the onion, celery and green pepper in preservative-free oil for about 5 minutes or until tender-crisp. Mix together the reserved juice, soya sauce, vinegar, brown sugar and flour. Stir into vegetables. Cook until thickened, stirring constantly. Stir in turkey and reserved peaches. Cook until heated through.

Yield: 4 servings

Veal Stew (Day 14)

1 tbsp	preservative-free oil	15 mL
¼ cup	chopped onion	50 mL
1	clove garlic, chopped fine or pressed	1
2 lb	stewing veal, cubed	1 kg
1 tsp	salt	5 mL
¼ tsp	pepper	1 mL
½ tsp	oregano	2 mL
1 tbsp	untreated white flour	15 mL
¾ cup	sliced celery	175 mL
2	large carrots, scraped and sliced	2
4	medium potatoes, peeled and quartered	4
2½ cups	hot water	625 mL

10 oz	frozen green beans	375 g

Heat preservative-free oil in a heavy casserole dish, and sauté onion and garlic for 5 minutes. Add veal, sprinkled with salt, pepper, oregano and flour. Toss and heat until the flour disappears. Add celery, carrots, potatoes and water. Simmer for 1 hour or until meat is tender. Add green beans, bring to a simmer and cook 5 minutes longer.

Yield: 6 servings of approximately 10 oz (375 g)

VEGETABLES

Stir-Fried Carrots, Peppers and Onions (Day 1)

2 tbsp	preservative-free oil	25 mL
4	carrots, sliced diagonally, ⅛ inch (3 mm) slices	4
1	green pepper, sliced, ⅛ inch (3 mm) slivers	1
1	green onions, cut in ½ inch (1 cm) slices	1 bunch
¼ cup	hot water	50 mL
¼ tsp	salt	1 mL
½ tsp	white sugar	2 mL

Set a heavy skillet over moderately high heat for 30 seconds. Add oil and swirl in pan. Heat for another 30 seconds. Add vegetables and stir constantly for 1 minute. Then add hot water, salt and sugar. Stir, cover and let steam for 2 minutes. Remove from heat and serve immediately.

Yield: 4 servings

Brown Rice (Days 1, 10, 13)

1 cup	brown rice	250 mL
2 cups	water	500 mL
1 tsp	salt	5 mL

Combine all ingredients in a saucepan. Bring to a boil and simmer until light and fluffy. At sea level follow package instructions. At high altitude brown rice can take up to an hour to cook.

Note: Rice retains more of its nutrients if it is not washed.

Yield: 4 servings

Sweet Potato Casserole (Day 2)

3 lb	sweet potato (1 large)	1.5 kg
19 oz	can unsweetened crushed pineapple	540 mL

Bake sweet potato, peel and whip. There should be approximately twice as much whipped potato as pineapple. Add pineapple, mix well and reheat.

Yield: Approximately 6 cups (1.5 L)

Oven French Fries (Days 3, 5)

4	medium to large potatoes	4
2 tbsp	preservative-free oil	25 mL
2 tbsp	water	25 mL

Scrub and peel potatoes or leave peel on if desired. Cut into matchsticks approximately ¼ inch (5 mm) thick. Mix oil and water well, and toss with the potatoes. Put potatoes on a cookie sheet greased with preservative-free oil. Bake for approximately 30 minutes at 450°F (230°C). Turn the strips after 15 minutes to brown evenly. If they don't brown well, brown under the broiler for a few minutes, but watch them carefully!

Yield: 4 servings

Beanpot Baked Lentils (Day 3)

1 cup	brown lentils	250 mL
½ cup	chopped onion	125 mL
2½ cups	water	625 mL
½ tsp	salt	2 mL
2 tbsp	brown sugar	25 mL
2 tbsp	Rhubarb Ketchup*	25 mL
2 tbsp	molasses	25 mL
½ tsp	dry mustard	2 mL

Rinse and drain the lentils. In a saucepan, combine the lentils, onion, water and salt. Bring to a boil. Cover and simmer for 1½ hours. Stir in remaining ingredients. Simmer in the saucepan or bake in a beanpot in a 350°F (180°C) oven for 1 hour (1½ -2 hours at high altitude) until tender and browned.

Yield: 4 servings

Funny Sort of Scalloped Potatoes (Day 4)

6	medium potatoes, sliced thin	6
2	medium onions, sliced thin	2
2 tbsp	minced parsley	25 mL
½ tsp	salt	2 mL
	freshly ground pepper	
3 tbsp	uncolored butter	45 mL
1½ cups	boiling water	375 mL

Preheat the oven to 400°F (200°C). Butter a shallow baking dish. Combine potatoes, onions, parsley, salt and pepper in the dish. Toss and spread evenly. Dot with butter. Pour boiling water over all. Bake for approximately 1 hour or until the water is absorbed and the potatoes are moist and tender but well browned on top.

Yield: 4-6 servings

Foil-Wrapped Potatoes and Onions (Day 7)

4	potatoes, peeled and cut in 5 slices	4
4	onions, peeled and cut in 4 slices	4
4 tsp	uncolored butter	20 mL
	Salt and pepper to taste	

On 4 pieces of heavy-duty foil, alternate slices of potato and onion. Dot with butter and sprinkle with salt and pepper. Seal foil well and bake for 1 hour at 400°F (200°C).

Yield: 4 servings

Hobo Vegetables (Day 8)

4	carrots, scraped	4
4	onions, peeled	4
4	potatoes, scrubbed	4
8 tsp	uncolored butter	40 mL
	Salt and pepper to taste	

Place a carrot, onion and potato on each of 4 pieces of heavy-duty foil. Add 2 tsp (10 mL) of butter and salt and pepper to each packet. Seal well and bake at 400°F (200°C) for 1 hour.

Note: These barbecue well. (Barbecue for approximately the same time.)

Yield: 4 servings

DESSERTS

Instant Fruit Sherbet (Day 1)

Take one can of unsweetened pears, peaches, pineapple, apricots, cherries or other berries in juice. Freeze the unopened can for 2-3 hours or until frozen. Run under hot running water for 1 minute. Open the can. Place chunks in a blender or food processor. Process until of sherbet consistency. Serve immediately.

Yield: 4 servings

Banana Sherbet (Day 6)

2	large bananas	2
¼ cup	pure lemon juice	50 mL
14 oz	can unsweetened pineapple	398 mL
½	can frozen raspberry juice concentrate	½

Purée all ingredients in a blender or food processor. Freeze until mushy; whip again and freeze.

Yield: 3½ cups (850 mL) sherbet

Jellied Fruit (Day 8)

½ cup	boiling water	125 mL
1½ cups	acceptable unsweetened fruit juice	375 mL
1 tbsp	unflavored gelatin	15 mL
1 cup	acceptable unsweetened diced fruit	250 mL
¼ cup	sunflower or sesame seeds	50 mL

Melt the gelatin in juice. Add boiling water and stir. Chill until slightly thickened. Fold in fruit and seeds. Chill to set.

Yield: 4 servings

BAKING

Whole Wheat Breadstick Worms (Days 6, 8)

3 cups	untreated whole wheat flour	750 mL
½ cup	wheat bran	125 mL
1 pkg	active dry yeast	1 pkg
½ tsp	salt	2 mL
1¼ cups	water	300 mL
¼ cup	uncolored butter	50 mL
2 tbsp	honey	25 mL
½ cup	sunflower seeds	125 mL
1	egg yolk	1
1 tbsp	water	15 mL

In a large bowl, stir together 2 cups (500 mL) of flour, the bran, yeast and salt. In a saucepan, heat water, butter and honey over low heat until warm. Gradually add to the dry ingredients, and beat at medium speed for 2 minutes. Add extra flour to make a soft dough. Beat for 2 minutes more at medium speed. Knead on a lightly floured board for 8-10 minutes until smooth and elastic. Knead in sunflower seeds. Put in a greased bowl, turning to grease all surfaces. Cover and let rise for 40 minutes.

Divide dough in half, rolling each half into a log shape. Cut each log into 12 pieces, shaping each piece into a 8-inch (20-cm) rope or "worm." Place on greased cookie sheets approximately 2 inches (5 cm) apart. Press in sunflower seeds for eyes! Cover and let rise for 30 minutes.

Mix together the egg yolk and 1 tbsp (15 mL) water. Brush ropes with the mixture and bake at 400°F (200°C) for 15 minutes. Cool on a wire rack.

Yield: 24 breadsticks

Hot Casserole Bread (Day 14)

1 pkg	active dry yeast	1 pkg
1 cup	warm water	250 mL
3¾ cups	untreated white flour	925 mL
1 tbsp	white sugar	15 mL

½ tsp	salt	2 mL
¼ -½ cup	extra water	50-125 mL
	uncolored butter to grease casseroles	

Soften 1 pkg of yeast in 1 cup (250 mL) of warm water. Measure flour into a bowl, and add the sugar and salt. Add water and yeast mixture and mix together. Stirring well, add enough extra water to make a soft dough. Cover and allow to rise until doubled in bulk.

Beat down the dough and put into a 1 qt (1 L) round, glass casserole dish that has been generously buttered. Allow to rise again until doubled in bulk.

Bake loaf in a 400°F (200°C) oven for 40 minutes. Remove from the casserole, and brush the crust with butter.

Note: Recipe can be doubled easily.

Yield: 1 loaf

BREAKFAST DISHES

Oatmeal (Days 2, 5, 9)

2 cups	water	500 mL
1 cup	quick-cooking rolled oats	250 mL

Bring the water to a boil, and stir in the oats. Lower heat, cover and simmer for 3-5 minutes. You can quickly get used to not having salt in cereal!

Yield: 4 servings

French Toast (Day 14)

1	egg	1
1 tsp	water	5 mL
	Dash of cinnamon	
	Few drops of vanilla	
1	slice milk-free whole wheat bread	1
2 tsp	uncolored butter	10 mL

Mix the first 4 ingredients. Soak the bread in the mixture until all of it is absorbed. Melt butter in a small frying pan, and brown the bread on one side. Turn and brown on the other side. Serve with Honey-Maple Syrup.*

Yield: 1 serving

SNACKS

Tropicalsicles (Day 3)
Purée 1 cup (250 mL) of canned unsweetened pineapple and 1 large banana. Pour into 8 popsicle makers.

Yield: 8 popsicles

Chick Dip (Day 6)

1½ cups	canned chickpeas, drained	375 mL
2	cloves garlic, minced	2
3 tbsp	pure lemon juice	45 mL
¼ cup	sesame seeds	50 mL
2 tbsp	chopped parsley	25 mL
	Salt and pepper to taste	

Purée all ingredients in a blender. If too stiff, add a little of the liquid from the chickpeas.

Yield: 1½ cups (375 mL)

Peanutsicles (Day 7)
Purée 2 small bananas or 1 medium with 2 tbsp (25 mL) of peanut butter. Pour into 4 popsicle makers.

Yield: 4 popsicles

Kids' Guacamole Dip (Day 9)

2	ripe avocados, peeled and diced	2
2 tsp	pure lemon juice	10 mL
2	cloves of garlic, minced	2
2	small onions, minced	2
½ tsp	salt	2 mL

Place all ingredients in a blender and whirl until puréed. Add more lemon if desired.

Yield: Approximately 1 cup (250 mL)

Potato-Skin Crisps (Day 13)

With kitchen shears cut leftover, baked potato skins into strips or small squares. Place skin-side-down in a single layer on a baking sheet and brush the inside of the skins with melted butter. Sprinkle with salt, pepper and garlic powder. Bake at 350°F (180°C) for 15 to 20 minutes until the skins are brown and crisp.

Yield: 1 serving per potato skin

Dandy Bean Dip (Day 14)

1 cup	dried red kidney beans	250 mL
2½ cups	water	625 mL
1	small onion, chopped	1
1-2	dried red chili peppers	1-2
¾ tsp	cumin	3 mL
1	clove garlic, minced	1
½ tsp	oregano	2 mL
¼ tsp	salt	1 mL

Combine all ingredients in a saucepan. Cover and bring to a boil. Reduce heat and simmer for 2½ hours (less time at sea level), or until beans are tender.

Drain and reserve cooking liquid. Blend the mixture in a food processor or blender. Gradually add cooking liquid until mixture has the consistency of a dip. A large can 28 oz (796 mL) of kidney beans can be substituted for cooked, dried beans.

Yield: 2 cups (500 mL)

Snow Cone (Day 14)

4	ice cubes	4
1 tsp	frozen fruit juice concentrate	15 mL

Crush 4 ice cubes in a blender or ice crusher, or place ice cubes in a plastic bag and crush with a hammer or wooden rolling pin. Pour the crushed ice into a small cup, and pour the thawed frozen fruit juice concentrate over the ice.

Yield: 1 serving

DRINKS

Jungle Juice (Days 7, 8)

Mix together 1 can of frozen blueberry juice concentrate (Westvale is a good brand), 1 can of acceptable frozen lemonade and 12 cans water. Mix well.

Green Giant Drink (Days 9, 10)

1 can	frozen lemonade concentrate	1
1 can	frozen limeade concentrate	1
12 cans	water	12

Mix concentrates and water together. As the yield is large (almost 4 qt/ 5 L) if the large cans of frozen juice are used, either small cans or a half recipe with the large cans may be more suitable for a small family.

Pink Drink (Days 11, 12)

⅓ can	frozen cranberry cocktail concentrate	⅓
1 can	frozen lemonade concentrate	1
8 cans	water	8

Mix ingredients together well. As with the Green Giant Drink, a half recipe may be more appropriate for a small family.

Fruit Drink (Days 13, 14)

1 part	normal dilution pineapple juice	1
1 part	normal dilution grapefruit juice	1
2 parts	water	2

Mix ingredients together well. Dole has a frozen pineapple-grapefruit concentrate which could be substituted for the fruit drink recipe. Add six cans of water to the concentrate instead of three cans.

Parsley Surprise (Day 14)

A Louise Lambert-Lagacé adaptation.

Place in a blender: ½ cup (125 mL) parsley, 1 cup (250 mL) unsweetened pineapple juice and a few ice cubes. Whirl.

Carrot-Pineapple Cocktail (Day 10)

A Louise Lambert-Lagacé adaptation.

Whirl in a blender: 2 cups (500 mL) unsweetened pineapple juice, 2 medium carrots and a ¼ -inch (5-mm) slice of lemon. Add 1 cup (250 mL) crushed ice, and whirl again.

ALTERNATE RECIPES

SOUPS

Basic Potato Soup

2 tbsp	preservative-free oil	25 mL
3	small onions, chopped	3
4	large potatoes, peeled and quartered	4
1 tsp	salt	5 mL
1	egg	1
	Chopped parsley or chives for garnish	

Heat oil and sauté onions until limp, not brown. Add potatoes, 6 cups (1.5 L) of water and salt. Cook for approximately 20 minutes or until the potatoes are tender. Whirl in a blender or food processor. Beat egg, and add a little hot soup to the egg. Add this mixture to the soup. Serve hot or cold with chopped parsley or chives. Other vegetables can be added to make carrot, broccoli or pea soups.

Yield: 6-8 servings

MAIN COURSE DISHES

Veal Patties

1	egg	1
2 tbsp	bread crumbs	25 mL
1 tsp	lemon peel, grated	5 mL
1 tsp	pure lemon juice	5 mL
½ tsp	salt	2 mL
	Pepper to taste	
3	green onions, chopped	3
1 lb	ground veal	500 g

In a large bowl, mix all ingredients together well except the onions and veal. Then mix in the veal and onions. Shape into 4-6 patties. Broil, barbecue, sauté or bake the patties.

Yield: 4-6 servings

Cold Meatloaf

1 lb	lean ground beef	500 g
½ lb	lean ground pork	250 g
2 cups	soft milk-free bread crumbs	500 mL
1 cup	water or vegetable water	250 mL
1	egg	1
¼ cup	onion, finely chopped	50 mL
1	clove garlic, crushed	1
½ tsp	salt	2 mL
¼ tsp	pepper	1 mL
¼ tsp	dry mustard	1 mL
¼ tsp	sage	1 mL
1 tbsp	pure horseradish	15 mL
2 tbsp	Rhubarb ketchup*	25 mL

Heat oven to 350°F (180°C). Combine meat and bread crumbs in a large bowl. In a separate bowl, beat water and egg together with a fork, and add to the meat mixture along with the remaining ingredients. Blend well with a fork, and pack into a loaf pan—preferably a glass pan. Bake for 1 ½ hours.

Drain off any liquid in the pan, and cool the meatloaf. Cover with foil or clear plastic wrap and chill. Makes an excellent cold meat for sandwiches. While chilling, try weighing down the loaf with a brick.

Yield: Approximately 18 slices

BAKING

Spicy Currant Cookies

½ cup	uncolored butter	125 mL
½ cup	brown sugar	125 mL
1	egg	1
1 tsp	pure vanilla extract	5 mL

1	infant prunes	1 jar
1 cup	untreated whole wheat flour	250 mL
1 tsp	baking powder	5 mL
1 cup	recommended infant cereal	250 mL
1 cup	dried currants	250 mL

In a large bowl, cream the butter and add the sugar. Beat until smooth. Add the egg, vanilla and prunes. In another bowl, stir flour, baking powder and infant cereal together, and mix well with the first mixture. Stir in the currants. Drop by the spoonful onto a cookie sheet greased with preservative-free oil. Press down with a fork moistened with water. Bake at 350°F (180°C) for 15-20 minutes or until done.

Yield: 24 cookies

Double Chocolate (Carob) Cookies

½ cup	uncolored butter	125 mL
¼ cup	brown sugar	50 mL
¼ cup	molasses	50 mL
1	egg	1
1 tsp	pure vanilla extract	5 mL
1	infant prunes	1 jar
1 cup	untreated whole wheat flour	250 mL
1 tsp	baking powder	5 mL
¼ cup	carob powder	50 mL
1½ cups	recommended infant cereal	375 mL
1 cup	milk-free carob chips	250 mL

In a large bowl, cream butter, and add sugar and molasses. Beat until smooth. Add egg, vanilla and prunes. Mix well. Sift flour, baking powder and carob powder together. Then add it to the butter mixture. Mix in infant cereal and carob chips. Drop by the spoonful onto a cookie sheet greased with preservative-free oil. Press down with a fork moistened with water. Bake at 350°F (180°C) for 16 minutes or until done.

Yield: 24 cookies

Carob Chip and Sunflower Seed Bars

| ½ cup | uncolored butter | 125 mL |
| ¾ cup | brown sugar, firmly packed | 175 mL |

1 tsp	pure vanilla extract	5 mL
2	eggs	2
1½ tsp	baking powder	7 mL
1½ cups	untreated whole wheat flour	375 mL
½ tsp	salt	2 mL
1 cup	milk-free carob chips	250 mL
1 cup	sunflower seeds	250 mL

Melt butter in a large saucepan. Remove from heat. Add sugar and vanilla, and stir until well blended. Add eggs one at a time, blending well after each addition. Mix together the flour, baking powder and salt. Add to saucepan and mix well. Spread evenly on a well-buttered 18 × 12-inch (45 × 30-cm) cookie sheet with rolled up edges. Sprinkle carob chips and sunflower seeds over the surface, and press them in lightly. Bake in a preheated oven at 350°F (180°C) for 30 minutes or until lightly browned. Cut into 2-inch (5-cm) squares while still warm.

Yield: 54 cookies

Pineapple Muffins

1	egg	1
1¼ cups	pineapple juice	300 mL
¼ cup	honey	50 mL
2 tbsp	preservative-free oil	25 mL
¾ cup	crushed unsweetened pineapple	175 mL
1¼ cups	bran	300 mL
½ cup	wheat germ	125 mL
1 cup	untreated whole wheat flour	250 mL
1 tsp	baking powder	5 mL
¼ tsp	salt	1 mL
1 cup	recommended infant cereal	250 mL

Preheat oven to 400°F (200°C), and grease 12 muffin tins with preservative-free oil. In a large bowl, beat the egg, and mix in the juice, honey and oil. Stir in pineapple, bran and wheat germ. In a separate bowl, mix flour, baking soda, salt and infant cereal. Add flour mixture to first mixture, stirring until just blended. Divide mixture evenly in muffin tins. Bake for 20-25 minutes until muffins are well browned and the tops spring back when touched lightly.

Yield: 12 muffins

Breakfast Bread

½ cup	untreated white flour	125 mL
1 cup	untreated whole wheat flour	250 mL
3 cups	recommended infant cereal	750 mL
½ tsp	baking soda	2 mL
2 tsp	baking powder	10 mL
⅓ cup	wheat germ	75 mL
¼ cup	brown sugar, firmly packed	50 mL
½ tsp	salt	2 mL
¼ cup	sesame seeds	50 mL
½ cup	untreated peanuts	125 mL
½ cup	dried currants	125 mL
3	eggs	3
½ cup	preservative-free oil	125 mL
½ cup	molasses	125 mL
¾ cup	pineapple juice	175 mL
1 cup	bananas, mashed	250 mL
⅓ cup	dried apricots, chopped	75 mL

Preheat oven to 325°F, (160°C) and grease 2 loaf pans with preservative-free oil. In a large bowl, mix the first 11 ingredients and blend well. In a blender, mix together the eggs, oil, molasses, juice and bananas. Add apricots, and whirl just long enough to chop apricots coarsely. Stir together wet and dry ingredients just until flour is moistened. Divide mixture evenly between the 2 loaf pans. Bake for approximately 1 hour or until the center is firm when lightly pressed with a fingertip. Cool slightly on a wire rack before removing from the pans. Cool completely before slicing.

Yield: 2 loaves, each 18 slices

No-Knead Health Bread

2 tsp	honey	10 mL
⅔ cup	lukewarm water	150 mL
2 pkg	dry active yeast	2 pkg
2 cups	lukewarm water	500 mL
3 tbsp	molasses	45 mL
5 cups	untreated whole wheat flour	1.25 L

½ tsp	salt	2 mL
⅓ cup	wheat germ	75 mL
⅓ cup	sesame seeds	75 mL

In a large bowl stir together the honey and ⅔ cup (150 mL) water. Add the yeast, stir and leave for 10 minutes until bubbly.

Combine 2 cups (500 mL) water and the molasses and add to the yeast mixture. Then add the flour, salt, wheat germ and seeds. Stir well. The dough will be sticky. Smooth into 2 loaf pans, well greased with preservative-free oil. Let the dough rise to the top of the pans. This usually takes about 1 hour.

Heat oven to 400°F, (200°C) and bake the bread for 30-35 minutes. Let the loaves cool in their pans on a wire rack. This is a heavy bread that is good for sandwiches, and it makes excellent toast.

Yield: 2 loaves, each 18 slices

No-Knead Oatmeal Bread

2 cups	boiling water	500 mL
1 cup	rolled oats	250 mL
1 tsp	white sugar	5 mL
⅔ cup	lukewarm water	150 mL
2 pkg	active dry yeast	½ pkg
½ cup	molasses	125 mL
½ tsp	salt	2 mL
1 tbsp	preservative-free oil	15 mL
5 cups	untreated whole wheat flour	1.25 L

Pour boiling water over the oats, and let them stand for 1 hour.

In a large bowl, dissolve the sugar in the lukewarm water, sprinkle the yeast on top and let stand for 10 minutes or until dissolved. Stir yeast and add to the oats. Add molasses, salt and oil. Gradually beat in the flour, working the last of the flour in with your hands. Shape into a ball, and place in a large greased bowl. Cover and let rise until it has doubled in size. This takes about 1 hour.

Punch down the dough, divide it in half and place in 2 bread pans greased with preservative-free oil. Smooth tops with a floured hand. Cover and let rise again until doubled in size, about 40 minutes. Bake in a 375°F (190°C) oven for 40-45 minutes. Remove from pans, and cool on racks.

Yield: 2 loaves

Wacky Carob Cake

1½ cup	untreated whole wheat flour	375 mL
1 tsp	baking soda	5 mL
½ tsp	salt	2 mL
⅓ cup	carob powder	75 mL
1 tsp	pure vanilla extract	5 mL
1 tsp	white vinegar	5 mL
⅓ cup	preservative-free oil	75 mL
⅓ cup	honey	75 mL
1 cup	water	250 mL

Preheat the oven to 350°F (180°C). In an ungreased pan, combine the dry ingredients. In a bowl, combine the vanilla, vinegar, oil, honey and water. Blend this into the dry mixture with a fork. Make sure that all the flour is mixed in. Bake for 25-30 minutes or until an uncolored toothpick inserted in the center comes out clean. Cool on a wire rack. When cool, cut into 16 2-inch (5-cm) squares.

Yield: 16 servings

DIET TIPS

Quick Banana Dog
Spread one split hot dog bun with peanut butter. Tuck in an entire peeled banana. This makes a popular lunch or breakfast.

What! No Gum?
Youngsters used to munching on gum can often be satisfied if given a small piece of honey comb to chew. Do make sure that they clean their teeth thoroughly after they are finished.

Mung Beans
One of the best ways to encourage youngsters to eat greens is to let them grow some. The popular mung bean

produces a sweet and tender sprout. Other mixed seeds and beans that can be purchased for sprouting are often too strong in flavor for kids.

Dippy Fruit
Provide child with a small plate covered, with a variety of fruit pieces and three small paper cups or egg cups. In one cup place a small amount of fruit juice. In the other two cups place homemade granola, coconut, toasted wheat germ or toasted sesame seeds. With an uncolored toothpick or cocktail fork, the child can spear the fruit, dip it in the juice and then in the variety of toppings.

Lettuce Rollups
Have your child wash a lettuce leaf and dry it with a towel. With a blunt knife, the child can spread the lettuce leaf with peanut butter or another nut butter such as sesame, cashew or almond butter. The child can then roll up the lettuce into a hot dog shape and eat it.

Coconut Chips
Drill holes in a fresh coconut and remove the milk. Bake the coconut at 425°F (220°C) for approximately 10 minutes, or until the shell cracks. Break it open, and let it cool. Let oven cool to 350°F (180°C).

In the meantime, remove the coconut meat from the shell, and remove the brown coating from the meat. With a potato peeler slice the coconut into paper-thin chips. Spread in one layer on a shallow baking pan, and sprinkle with salt. Stir the coconut occasionally while baking. Cook for approximately 30 minutes, or until brown and crisp. Cool to room temperature, and keep in a tightly covered container.

CHAPTER EIGHT

COPING WITH FINICKY EATERS

Whenever our son wants a food he can't have, he says, "I'm sick and tired of them putting MSG in all this food." Whenever he doesn't want a particular food, he says, "I can't have that, I'm allergic."

—MOTHER OF A SIX-YEAR-OLD HYPERACTIVE BOY

AT THE BEST OF TIMES, small people rebel and can be utterly exasperating when it comes to mealtime. When major changes are made in their diets, they are likely to protest loudly. However, there are many strategies that will help you cope with them.

MEALTIME STRATEGIES

Portion Size

Keep it small. Babies eat and eat because they are growing so quickly. As growth levels off, there is a sudden drop in appetite. No child is deliberately going to starve, and we do tend to underestimate the amount they actually eat. Pint-sized people require only pint-sized portions. How would you like to have your meal served on a large platter and have it consist of a whole roast chicken with 2 cups of gravy, 2 lbs of mashed potatoes, 2 lbs of diced carrots, 2 lbs of peas and a dozen buttered buns? And be told to eat every mouthful? Wouldn't your appetite quickly fade as theirs undoubtedly does when they are given disproportionately large servings?

Like Parent Like Child

Although children will have food preferences that are not identical to those of Mom and Dad, they do tend to mimic their parents. If Dad is enjoying his pretzels and beer, there is no way that junior is going to be bought off with a carrot. If Mom doesn't eat her vegetables, it is highly unlikely that her children will eat theirs.

If it is possible for the entire family to participate in this food experiment, you will have far fewer problems than if your child is expected to eat one meal while the rest of the family is eating something else (especially if the something else is a favorite food). When other family members just have to have a non-diet food fix, be sure they have it outside the home or after the little one is sound asleep. Parents also need a little change from time to time. If during these trials you can find a competent babysitter who will not sabotage the diet, give yourselves a break and go out and have a nice restaurant meal. However, if you are following the diet and experimenting with your own reactions to food, be careful about what you order. Usually a barbecued steak without sauce, a baked potato and a salad with lemon or oil and vinegar is a fairly safe bet. Keep in mind that alcohol (even a little) contains many additives.

Fun with Food

Balky eaters are much more likely to eat the foods that they help prepare than those that are just presented to them. If you let your child roll out breadsticks ("worms"), help assemble a "mouse" salad, mix ingredients for gorp or whirl a slurpee (with supervision), he'll feel in control of the situation. You'll also be instilling in him good diet habits, which is a bonus. And who knows, your child might become a famous chef!

Be Flexible

If your child wants to eat out of the baby's dish, why not? If the dog's dish is today's favorite plate, run it through the dishwasher first. Most young children love to eat from zany utensils. They also love foods they can eat with their fingers. There is no harm in indulging these sorts of whims.

Mealtime Is a Nice Time

Mealtime should be a family affair. Encourage chatting and sharing, not grumbles and battles.

I Won't Eat It

It's important not to overreact when children say they won't eat something. Kids love to refuse, tease and test to see what your limits are. You can either give in and run and individualized catering service, or you can be firm and say that this is what is being served at this meal. Don't beg your youngster to eat it. Say, "Try it, you might like it" or "This will make you run faster, jump higher, see like a cat, or roar like a lion." Or you can use the strategy that I used for years, which still sends my children into great gales of laughter. I would say, "This is a new food, very expensive and I only got enough for Daddy and me." Or "This is pretty strong, spicy, exotic." Or "I think you're too little, too young, wouldn't appreciate it." Or the real clincher, "It's grown-up food." It worked every time.

As well, for years we had a really proper dinner on Sunday evenings with candlelight, a special tablecloth and the good china. Quite often I would introduce a new food at these dinners, and the kids wouldn't act up while they were having such a terribly grown-up experience. At one of these dinners, our son, then six, announced that when he grew up he was going to have chateaubriand garni, sauce béarnaise and a really good bottle of red wine every night for dinner. (He doesn't.)

Also, do listen to what your child is saying about a particular food. Young children have a keener sense of smell and more sensitive taste buds than adults; consequently, they may be more aware of foods that have an "off" flavor.

Sweets

Parents are largely responsible when a child develops a sweet tooth, not the child. Children who are not introduced to very sweet foods or trained to believe sweets are best seldom miss them. The recipes provided in this book have a much lower sugar content than most recipes. Our experience has shown that once the kids have eaten foods made from these recipes for a period of time, they actually prefer them.

You will notice that there are a variety of cookies, muffins and slushes in the recipe chapter. If all these "fun" items are removed from children's diets, they will rebel, because it is very important for them to be like other kids. Moderation and adaptation are the key things to remember when your child asks for sweets.

Distractions and Dawdling

Children know that there are many more more exciting things to do than eat, such as watching TV, playing with toys and so on. You will get better cooperation if a meal is served at the table away from such distractions. At the table, be aware of the child's pace of eating, not yours. He or she may be overtired, may hate the food or may simply not be hungry. There is no sense in keeping a child at the table for extended periods of time if he or she isn't up to finishing a meal. Table time should be limited to fifteen to twenty minutes.

Ants in Pants at the Table

Parents of very hyperactive children are often frustrated not by dawdling but by their youngster's inability to stay still at the table. Such children will often engage in repetitive table leg banging, foot stamping, finger tapping and so on. In many cases, having a few minutes' quiet time just prior to a meal can help, as can requiring the child to stay at the table only for the main course, then it's up, up and away with a low-sugar cookie or a piece of fruit.

BEGGING FOOD FROM RELATIVES AND NEIGHBORS

SOME WELL-MEANING grandparents can interfere with their grandchildren's diets, as they simply cannot believe that their little dimpled darling is a problem. In order to prove the point, some parents have been known to load their youngsters with junk food prior to a visit with the grandparents to show how rotten the kids can be. More often than not, parents know what wires their child—at least they know what some of the trigger items are—and they normally avoid these items. Often, however, when the youngster goes visiting, the treats are the taboo items. And, frequently, there is a delayed reaction to these items, which does not occur until the child returns home.

The best way to handle interfering relatives or friends is to be firm with them and at the same time to encourage them to participate in making special foods for your child. Either take allowed treats with you when you visit them and let them dole out the treats, or get them involved in preparing special cookies or treats. As a last resort, if all else fails, avoid visiting the uncooperative relative or friend while you are carrying out the initial diet test.

You will find the uncooperative friend or relative to be the exception; most people, including many grandparents, will be very cooperative. They will check with you before feeding the child or ask to be provided with appropriate meals or snacks. Some parents type up lists of appropriate foods. You will find that many of your friends with children are very nutrition-conscious and will welcome the opportunity to try some of your new recipes and ideas.

CHAPTER NINE

WHAT TO FEED THEM WHEN THEY'RE SICK

In the year that followed the change in diet, he was on penicillin only twice, instead of the six times the previous year.
—MOTHER OF A HYPERACTIVE FIVE-YEAR-OLD BOY

YOU ARE LIKELY TO ENCOUNTER a sick day or two during the diet trial, so it is best to be prepared. If medication is required, ask your physician to prescribe drugs which are not artificially colored or flavored; for example, white Tylenol tablets or white penicillin tablets. For those allergic to penicillin, some physicians have prescribed Ilosone (Erythromycin Estolate) removed from its capsule and dissolved in water. I'm told the taste is not unpleasant.

Your little patient is more likely to cooperate if you offer him or her a variety of foods and beverages. If he or she is only tolerating clear fluids, here are a few suggestions:

• Sparkling or plain mineral water, such as Canada Dry Sparkling Water or Shasta Club Soda
• Slightly flat regular gingerale or regular 7Up
• Regular-strength acceptable juices, such as Minute Maid Lemonade or Limeade, Ocean Spray Cranberry Cocktail. Dilute if regular-strength juice is not well tolerated, but regular strength will provide more food energy.

- Homemade beef or chicken broth
- Jelly made with plain gelatin and acceptable regular-strength juice
- Popsicles made with regular-strength acceptable juices

When your child is feeling a little better, add:

- Cooked pear, peach, apricot and raw banana fruit slurpees and sherbets
- Puréed homemade soups (use vegetables that don't produce gas when digested). Potato makes a good base for no-milk creamlike soups; potato plus carrots, asparagus or peas and so on.
- Fruit shakes

If tolerated, add:

- Plain cooked oatmeal or Cream of Wheat (no seeds or raisins)
- White toast
- White homemade melba toast
- Cooked tapioca with fruit juice
- Cooked fruit, vegetables and meat (avoid skins, seeds, herbs and spices)

Gradually add the foods that are normally eaten.

Beware of colored straws and other disposable paper goods. Plain, uncolored straws are available at many pharmacies. Now might be the time to buy your little one his or her own little bowl, mug and plate. Just make sure that the colors do not come off.

Humidifiers are fine, but some children have reacted to the medications that are used with them.

Cough medicines are usually colored and flavored and have been reported to cause dramatic behavior and sleep changes. Some parents have found that a fifty-fifty mixture of pure fresh lemon juice or frozen Minute Maid lemon juice and pure honey is useful. The following recipe may also prove effective.

Homemade Cough Medicine

¼ cup (50 mL) unsulphured molasses
1 tbsp (15 mL) uncolored butter
1 tbsp (15 mL) white vinegar
3 tbsp (45 mL) finely chopped onion

Boil all ingredients together for 5 minutes and then strain. Cool and give 1 tsp (5 mL) as necessary.

These suggestions are no substitute for your doctor's orders. Be sure to call your physician when your child is ill.

CHAPTER TEN

WORKING AROUND SPECIAL OCCASIONS

Our child is not now an easygoing personality, but when allergic reactions are not affecting him, he is "normal" in his behavior, and we all enjoy life together more.
—MOTHER OF A THREE-YEAR-OLD HYPERACTIVE BOY

IT'S A SNAP, or more or less a snap, to cope with a diet when nothing special is happening. However, it's a different story when your youngster has a birthday to celebrate, is invited to a birthday party or wants to graze with the other kids at sports events and movies. As well, we have the holidays to deal with. Here are just a few ideas that may save a little hair-pulling.

OTHER PEOPLE'S BIRTHDAY PARTIES

NOTHING IS MORE DEVASTATING for a child than not being permitted to go to a party. Usually, parents of the party child will be supportive of your child's special needs, if they do not cause any extra work for them. If the parents are willing to provide you with the menu, you can write a list for them of items tolerated on their menu and provide similar replacement items for the other foods and beverages; for example, additive-free wieners, additive-free potato chips, a little white homemade cupcake with white icing decorated with pure gummy bears made from fruit juice, a good fruit punch made from tolerated juices, additive-free buns and so on.

Restaurant birthday meals can be a little shakier, but most restaurants will reheat or chill homemade items. A visit or telephone call to the restaurant (during off-peak hours) prior to the occasion is a good idea. Often they will have special items which they can suggest preparing for your child. Many restaurants are becoming much more attuned to special diet needs.

YOUR CHILD'S BIRTHDAY PARTY

EVEN BEFORE I BEGAN to do research in the area of food allergy and intolerance, one of my joys as a mother was planning birthday parties for my little people. Here are some ideas I've used for special parties. The menus are all adaptable to special diet needs.

Red Riding Hood Party
This is ideal for two-to five-year-olds. Take your child's guests to a local park. Once you get there, provide each child with a homemade red cotton hooded cape and a little straw basket containing their own lunch. Some things you might consider putting in their baskets are: little party sandwiches, a pick-up-stick lunch, fruit, vegetable, meat or poultry kabobs, vegetables or fruit with dip, breadsticks or individual cupcakes. The take-home treat can be the hood, basket and napkin.

Hawaiian Luau
Good for school-aged children. Although ideal for a summer party around a pool, it can be held anytime indoors with a little imaginative decorating. Girls are each supplied with a simple, homemade flowered muumuu made from cheap gaudy cotton. Boys are provided with inexpensive tropical-style shirts. Food consists of huge platters of pineapple chunks, papaya chunks, banana slices

or other seasonal fruits, ham cubes and Chinese Chicken pieces, all speared with toothpicks. Buns or breadsticks can be provided. Dessert is assorted balls of fruit ices garnished with mint. Beverage is a fruit punch. We had hula hoop and dance contests, made paper leis and played Hawaiian music at our party. The take-home gift can be the muumuu or shirt and the lei.

Cinderella Party

This definitely has more appeal for young girls. Precut simple crowns and wands from stiff cardboard and provide each child with strips of aluminum foil, Scotch Tape, sequins and glue to complete their princess attire. Serve tiny crustless princess sandwiches (a real treat if they always have to eat their crusts), tiny vegetables and pumpkin cake. Children can play make-a-wish games, telling one another their most outrageous fantasies. The take-home gift can be the wand and crown.

Backwards Party

At this party for school-age children, guests are instructed to wear as many of their clothes backwards as they can. They try to walk backwards, say goodbye when they come instead of hello, eat immediately and play afterwards. At the birthday table, place the chairs backwards so that the kids have to kneel on them and eat over the backs. Serve dessert first. At our party, the children had so much fun working at doing everything backwards, eating with the wrong utensils and trying to talk backwards that they spent all their time at the table.

Hobo Party

My son's birthday is in November, sort of a dreary month for a birthday, and he bemoaned the fact that one of his sisters could always have her party out of doors in August, so we decided to have an outdoor party indoors. In the middle of the room, we prepared a circle of bright autumn leaves with a plate in the middle holding a can of Sterno. My son's friends were asked to come dressed as hobos. When they came to the kitchen to pick up their "hobo meal," they were given a long stick with a hobo bundle tied in a bright bandana. The bundle contained cold baked chicken, carrot sticks, potato chips and a cupcake. Beverages were served in washed-out tin cans. We lit the canned heat, turned down the lights to make the "campfire" look more authentic, and the youngsters told each other ghost stories. The take-home gift was their stick and bandana.

Fondue Party

This is a lot of fun for older children—a kind of glorified hamburger party with a twist. Serve tiny meatballs, which the kids can cook in a fondue pot with oil. Provide a variety of sauces, finger foods and crusty rolls as accompaniments. Dessert can be a fruit sauce fondue with appropriate fruit, cake and nut "dippers." You might want to serve beverages in wine or champagne glasses to make them look glamorous.

GRAZING

PARENTS HAVE COME UP with some ingenious ways to cope with those snacks after sports events and movies. Children who are normally intolerant of even moderate amounts of sugar appear to tolerate more when they are physically active. After the hockey or soccer game or while actively skiing, skating or participating in other demanding sports, a milk-free carob bar, pure fruit jellies, a can of regular 7Up or a can or bottle of regular-strength juice is better tolerated than during inactive periods.

Most families have found that in order to have their child sit through a full-length movie without an attack of "ants in the pants," they have to bring snacks and treats from home, such as diluted lemonade and additive-free potato chips. If you are far enough along with your diet and testing to have determined that corn is not a problem, consider bringing popcorn. Most parents have reported that their youngsters have coped better with homemade popcorn than the popcorn supplied in the theaters. Not quite so glamorous, but a reasonable substitute.

CHRISTMAS

CHRISTMAS MENUS CAN BE easily adapted to this diet. However, a few words of warning are in order. For some reason, children have had some of the most serious behavioral reactions to mandarin oranges from Japan. The mandarin oranges from California do not cause such reactions. Also, children who have allergies or intolerances can be intolerant of Christmas trees, either natural or artificial. Your local allergy association will have information on this subject.

EASTER

MOST CHILDREN ASSOCIATE Easter with chocolate. If you are fortunate enough to live in a community where the local candy shop makes carob candy, you will often find Easter carob bunnies and eggs. In another attempt to find a substitute for chocolate, some parents have organized penny hunts instead of Easter egg hunts. Some little girls like new Easter finery, such as a pretty dress, costume jewelry, or hair ornaments. Other children are not turned on by these and prefer new books or a fuzzy toy animal. We have put together some rather ingenious Easter baskets for them: a child's plastic hard hat can be filled with a variety of items, such as games, miniature cars, fuzzy bunnies and chickens, little books or comics, goggles or sunglasses or a magnifying glass. A much happier solution than an out-of-control space cadet!

KOSHER COOKING FOR FESTIVE OCCASIONS

SINCE MOST FOODS prepared for traditional Jewish holidays are made-from-scratch foods, adaptations for this diet have not been difficult for my patients. There have not been additives in any of the brands of matzoh or matzoh meal that I have seen. At Chanukah, pear sauce makes a good substitute for applesauce on potato latkes. Chopped dates can be substituted for raisins in most recipes, and grated or chopped firm pear substitutes nicely for apple. Honey cake and other sweets associated with celebrations need not be eliminated, merely eaten in moderation at the end of the meal. With the exclusion of milk and dairy products, additive-free soy products such as tofu or other pareve foods (permitted fish, eggs, fruit, vegetables) can be substituted. Parents concerned about the lack of protein in the milk-free diet need not worry unless the children do not eat meat or poultry. They will receive moderate amounts of protein from grains and vegetables, and the addition of a sprinkle of sesame seeds, sunflower seeds or an extra serving of gorp will boost their protein intake.

HALLOWEEN

THANK GOODNESS TRICK-OR-TREATING is not as popular as it once was. Many teachers and parents have reported that children are absolutely impossible to work and live with after both Halloween and Easter. Many communities, churches and other organizations are now having parties where there is less emphasis on candy. If there is nothing organized in your community, why not plan a party for your children and their friends? You might want to use some of the following suggestions:

• Bob for fall pears instead of apples.

• Create your own Spook House. Blindfold children, then

lead them through the ghoulish experience of feeling "eyeballs" (peeled grapes), "worms" (cold spaghetti) and "brains" (slightly stirred gelatin). Then have them walk on a partially inflated air mattress while spooky music plays. After everyone has gone through this experience, you can allow them to see what they have touched and walked on.

- If they insist upon going trick-or-treating, you might consider buying unsuitable treats for a penny an item, then taking the children to a senior citizens' home or center to distribute the goodies. Some parents purchase a few treats that their child does tolerate, such as Sorbee sugarless candies and lollipops, nuts in the shell and preservative-free pretzels or potato chips.
- Other possibilities in lieu of candies are stuffed animals, such as black cats, or well-washed orange and black balloons.
- My daughter, who teaches swimming, told me about another good idea. One of her young charges told her how lucky their family was on Halloween: the other kids went trick-or-treating for just one night. However, her parents had bought a twenty-night family pass to the pool, so she and her brother were getting much more than the other kids.
- Serving toasted pumpkin seeds can become a tradition at Halloween. After scooping out the seeds to make your jack-o'-lantern, wash the seeds and remove as many of the strings as possible. Soak the seeds in salted water overnight (½ tsp/2.5 mL salt to ½ cup/150 mL water). Place seeds on a cookie sheet in a 300°F (150°C) oven for 20 minutes or until golden. Salt to taste.
- For a special dessert, try a scoop of papaya or peach ice decorated with a carob chip or dried black currant face to resemble a jack-o'-lantern.
- And Pumpkin Bars are a nice treat anytime.

Pumpkin Bars

½ cup	preservative-free oil	125 mL
⅓ cup	honey	75 mL
2	eggs	2
1 cup	untreated whole wheat flour	275 mL
+ 2 tbsp		
1 tsp	baking powder	5 mL
½ tsp	baking soda	2 mL
1 cup	cooked mashed pumpkin	250 mL
¾ tsp	cinnamon	3 mL
⅓ cup	untreated, tolerated nuts or seeds	75 mL

In a bowl, mix all ingredients together. Spread on a 13 × 9 × 2-inch (33 × 25 × 5-cm) pan. Bake at 350°F (180°C) for 25-30 minutes. Cut into bars.

CHAPTER ELEVEN

REINTRODUCING PROBLEM FOODS

The "silly fits" are very diet related, and we are continuing to identify what causes them.

—MOTHER OF A THREE-YEAR-OLD GIRL

YOU HAVE JUST COMPLETED the first phase of the Hyperactivity Test Diet plan. For four weeks your family and child have followed the diet (with just the occasional noted slip), and you have kept a daily diary, noting your child's behavior, physical symptoms and sleep patterns. Now, it's time to play detective.

You may think you have seen a remarkable change; instead of an out-of-control little terror, you seem to have a pretty good kid. Unfortunately, some of you will feel there has been little change. This is where your daily diaries can help solve the puzzle. Get them out, then photocopy and fill in the chart that appears on the next page.

SUMMARY OF BEHAVIOR, SLEEP AND PHYSICAL SYMPTOMS

DAY	BEHAVIOR SCORE	SLEEP SCORE	PHYSICAL SCORE	SCORE TOTAL FOR DAY
1.				
2.				
3.				
4.				
5.				
6.				
7.				
8.				
9.				
10.				
11.				
12.				
13.				
14.				
15.				
16.				
17.				
18.				
19.				
20.				
21.				
22.				
23.				
24.				
25.				
26.				
27.				
28.				

Has the Score Total for the Day decreased significantly from Day 1 to Day 28?

If so, have the scores for individual items—behavior, sleep or physical symptoms—decreased significantly from Day 1 to Day 28?

If there is a significant decrease in one or more of the individual items, examine your daily records carefully. You can determine which characteristics have changed the most.

On a separate sheet of paper, list the three to five characteristics that are most improved. When you are reintroducing foods, you can watch for the possible return of these noted characteristics.

DECISIONS, DECISIONS, WHAT TO TRY

WHEN REINTRODUCING FOODS, common sense should prevail. If your child has had a severe reaction to a food in the past, obviously you shouldn't reintroduce even a tiny bit of it at home. Make an appointment with your physician for your youngster to be retested for the allergy or for the food to be given to him or her under medical supervision.

The next point to consider when reintroducing foods is good nutrition. Now that your child is eating a nutritious diet, which is low in sugar and high in complex carbohydrate and fiber, why not continue feeding him or her this way? If your whole family has participated in the diet and you are pleased with the change in life-style and the general feeling of well-being within the family, you may want to test only highly nutritious foods that have been removed from your diet for the trial. These include low-fat milk and dairy products, oranges, apples, tomatoes, corn, grapes, raisins and the more nutritious processed foods such as chunky soups.

In determining in what order to reintroduce food into your child's diet, you can let yourself be governed to some extent by his or her desires and by the availability of products. If your child craves apples, and is not making complaints that would lead you to suspect apples are a problem, then go ahead and test apple products. If there are no preservative-free breads available in your area, and you don't want to continue to bake bread, it would make sense to test for sensitivity to BHT and BHA. If your youngster does not react to these additives, you can once again use a commercial bread. However, if your child is begging to try colored jelly beans, think twice. Aside from the fact that these only provide empty calories, how are you going to tell, if your child reacts to them, whether the reaction is to sugar, color, flavor or the excitement of being able to have candy again?

It's important not to underestimate the excitement factor. If a child hasn't had a food or additive for a long time, and it is a favorite food, you may get a reaction simply because he or she is excited about having the food. As well, you may be watching the poor child so closely for a reaction that you may imagine one. The best way to handle reintroducing foods is to hide the food in another food. For example, you could test apple juice by adding it to cranberry juice or skim milk powder by putting it in baked goods or a casserole. By not telling the child what you are doing, you can eliminate the excitement factor.

If you want to be totally unbiased in your testing, you can involve a third person. Over a period of three to five designated testing days, that person either adds or does not add the test item to the meal. You still rate your child's behavior, sleep and physical symptoms. You are not told until after the tests are completed which meals contained the test item and which meals did not.

If your records show significant changes in any of the three areas under scrutiny when a test item was added to a meal, you have probably detected an offender. If the records do not show any changes, you can either retest or presume that the tested item is not an offender. Occasionally all this testing can be confusing, because there is the possibility of certain foods and/ or chemicals causing a reaction when they are combined. In scientific terms this is referred to as *synergistic effect*. To give you an example, say you have individually tested ketchup, mustard, green relish, regular hot dog buns and regular hot dogs. You have observed no reaction to the items when tested separately, but combined they may be like a stick of dynamite. It can happen.

It is also important not to attribute all behavioral reactions to food. For example, to start your son's day, you put his cereal in the wrong bowl. Then his older sister teases him all through breakfast. Later he learns that his playmate has a bad cold and isn't allowed to play outside. There are days like this, and it is impossible to attribute a temper tantrum after lunch on this kind of day to what your child ate. Do the test when all is well with the world.

If your records show no change, I suggest trying what my patients call "junk-loading". The idea is to reintroduce everything that has been eliminated within a twenty-four hour period. Foods and drinks for junk-loading include:

- A standard chocolate cake mix with canned frosting and colored sprinkles. This provides a sugar load, chocolate, artificial colors and probably BHT, BHA and caffeine.
- A frozen deluxe pizza. This provides tomato, cheese, added nitrates, MSG and BHT.
- Pure monosodium glutamate, seasoning salt.
- Regular cola, which provides sugar, caffeine, color and flavor.
- Powdered fruit-flavored drinks. These provide artificial color and flavor and sugar.

This may sound foolhardy after what I have previously said, but several children who showed marginal results during the test diet reacted strongly to the loading. Among their most pronounced symptoms were poor behavior and headaches. One little fellow, after four hours of junk-loading, went to his mother and said, "Please don't feed me this stuff anymore. I don't like me and nobody will play with me." He had also tripped down the stairs during this period and had been abnormally poorly coordinated. Although it may take a few hours or days for the effects to wear off, if the child is convinced that the type of foods he or she has been eating for the previous four weeks make him or her feel better, you have won the good nutrition battle. If there is no reaction to junk-loading, there is little or no reason to believe that foods, additives, food flavor enhancers or stimulants such as caffeine are affecting your child's behavior. However, a good healthy diet is still one of the greatest gifts you can give your child.

For those parents who appear to have had positive results from the test diet, patience is important. Although children may react almost immediately to a food, the reaction may not be obvious for several hours, and in some cases a few days. For this reason, it is necessary to reintroduce foods slowly and to be fairly sure that the test item in question is not causing a problem before going on to the next food. A good rule of thumb is one item per week. Of course, if a child continues to react to a food for several days, he or she should not be exposed to a new food until all symptoms have disappeared.

REINTRODUCING SPECIFIC FOODS

Milk and Dairy Products
If your child has exhibited physical symptoms commonly associated with milk allergy, reintroduce milk slowly and carefully.

DAY 1: Add 2 tsp (10 mL) skim milk powder to breakfast. If no reaction is observed,

Day 2: Add 2 tsp (10 mL) skim milk powder to breakfast and lunch.

If no reaction is observed,

Day 3: Add 2 tsp (10 mL) skim milk powder to each meal. Powder can be added to oatmeal, casseroles, soup, fruit drinks or popsicles.

If no reaction has been observed by the end of the third day, add other plain dairy products.

Day 4: Add plain yogurt, which can be dressed up with fruit or nuts, and cottage cheese, uncolored hard cheese such as cheddar and mozzarella.

Children who have previously been given excessive amounts of milk and dairy products, and who are not reacting to milk, should be restricted to 2 cups (500 mL) per day. As a dairy substitute you can give them 3 oz (90 g) of natural hard cheese or 1½ cups (375 mL) of yogurt. Each of these will provide approximately 600 mg of calcium. If your child tolerates this amount of milk and dairy products, you can discontinue giving him or her calcium and vitamin D supplements. If your child will not drink milk, but is getting an equivalent amount from other dairy products, you can discontinue using calcium; however, continue with vitamin D during the cold months.

If your child displays reactions to milk—bad breath, stomachaches, runny nose, congestion, rashes—talk to your physician or dietitian. He or she will be able to determine whether the reaction is a milk-sugar (lactose) intolerance or a milk-protein intolerance, and then provide you with appropriate counseling. It is also possible that excluding milk from your child's diet for four to six months may make him or her more tolerant. At the end of that time, I would advise giving the child a small amount of milk every three to four days to test tolerance, and gradually increasing the amount. It is important to retest for tolerance, several times if necessary, and not to permanently exclude nutritious foods unless absolutely necessary. Although they are unable to tolerate dairy products daily, many children are able to tolerate small servings once or twice a week.

Apple
When reintroducing, add a mixture of one part pure apple juice and one part water to raspberry juice or cranberry cocktail. If no reaction is noted after three days, add peeled apple sections. (Children have reacted to apple skins, especially bright red ones.) If there is no reaction, apple can be put back in the diet, but encourage the child to continue to eat and drink a variety of fruits and juices.

Grape and Raisin
First try white bottled grape juice, added as above to other juices. If well tolerated, try small portions of grapes, about ¼ cup (50 mL), or 1 tbsp (15 mL) sun-dried raisins (Sunmaid are good). If tolerated, keep portions small, because grapes and raisins contain significant amounts of natural sugars.

Orange
Test pure, unsweetened orange juice as above. If there is no reaction, try orange slices or sections. If there is a reaction to pre-prepared juice but not to oranges, the reaction could be to the oil from the orange skins or to other parts of the skin that have found their way into the juice during the mechanical squeezing process.

Tomato
Add tomato, pure tomato sauce, paste or juice to a meat or vegetable soup or stew. Many children tend to develop a red rash around their lips after eating tomato. Be sure to test tomato before testing tomato ketchup. There are several ingredients in ketchup which could cause reactions.

Corn

Add puréed canned corn to a soup or stew. If tolerated, try other forms of corn, such as canned or frozen kernels, corn on the cob, popcorn, cornstarch and corn syrup.

Sugar (Simple Sugars)

The purpose of this test is to determine the effect of refined carbohydrate and concentrated sources of natural sugars on your child. When testing sugar, use only foods on your product list and tested acceptable foods. Do not use high-sugar foods with added artificial colors and flavors.

For two days, this is the procedure to follow:

1. Restrict meat, eggs, peanut butter and dairy products, if tolerated, to recommended daily amounts.
2. Encourage your child to consume foods that are high in natural sugars; for example, honey, maple syrup, dates, figs and sweetened juices.
3. Encourage your child to also eat foods that are high in refined sugars; for example, sugar, corn syrup if tolerated, additive-restricted granola bars, pure jams, sesame snaps, high-sugar homemade cakes, cookies and pies.

If your child responds in a negative manner to this test (i.e., if he or she whines, is irritable, runs in circles, bites, kicks and so on), the experiment can be discontinued before the testing period is over.

Monosodium Glutamate

Among the most amusing stories are those which have to do with testing monosodium glutamate. Perhaps the winner was one from a greatly distressed mother who called to say, "I just tested him on MSG and he pulled down his pants and wagged it at me. Would MSG do that?" In my clinical practice we often do see bold, cheeky, aggressive or repetitive behavior when MSG is reintroduced into a child's diet.

To test your child's reaction to MSG, make homemade

soup or stew, reducing the normal amount of salt in the recipe by at least half. To the child's portion add ¼ tsp (1 mL) monosodium glutamate (one brand name is Accent). If your child does not react to this amount, at another meal try adding ½ tsp (2 mL). If your child tolerates MSG, you will be able to add many processed foods, seasoning salts, sauces and salad dressings to your larder. However, you will find that there are many other additives in most of these foods as well. You might also want to keep in mind that MSG and its kissing cousins, hydrolyzed plant protein (HPP) and hydrolyzed vegetable protein (HVP), have no nutritional value.

Benzoates
If your child tolerates 7Up, an easy way to test his or her tolerance for benzoates is to give him or her a small amount of Sprite (½ cup/125 mL). (Sprite and 7Up are similar, except that Sprite contains benzoates.) If your child cannot tolerate the amount of sugar contained in soft drinks, then use club soda or unsweetened pickles with benzoates for the test. Watch pickles for spices.

BHT and BHA
The easiest way to test BHT and BHA is with the pure chemical (for example, anti-oxidant BHT made by Twin-lab), adding just a sprinkle to a fruit slurpee or stew. Another possibility is to give your child Triscuits with 50 percent less salt. These contain only whole wheat, shortening (coconut or vegetable oil), salt and BHT in the packaging, which does permeate the food. Quaker Shredded Wheat contains only wheat and BHA. Nabisco Spoon-Sized Shredded Wheat, Nabisco Shredded Wheat, and Sunshine Shredded Wheat contain only wheat and BHT. It would not appear from clinical observations that a large number of people are intolerant of these preservatives, and if there is no intolerance, many crackers, cereals and other healthy foods can be reintroduced. BHT and BHA keep foods fresh and prevent rancidity; however,

there remains some controversy about their safety. My preference is to use additive-free breads and oils, but in order to provide variety, you may want to use crackers and cereals containing these substances.

Chocolate
Since most chocolate contains many ingredients other than chocolate, only the following should be used for testing purposes:

- Baker's Unsweetened Chocolate (100 percent pure chocolate).
- Baker's Sweetened Chocolate (contains sugar, chocolate, cocoa butter, butter oil, soy lecithin). Use only if your child can tolerate all the ingredients.
- Hershey's Cocoa (contains cocoa, sodium carbonate, salt).

If your child is intolerant of chocolate, it is quite possible that he or she will have an intolerance to cola as well. They are from the same botanical family, and there is often an intolerance to both.

Cola
Try Classic Coke for testing purposes. There are several other ingredients in colas which your child might react to. If there is no reaction, keep in mind that the fruit juices and fruit slurpees that your child has been having beat pop hands down in terms of nutritional value.

Caffeine
You may find that your youngster reacts to chocolate and cola, but not to tea and coffee. As mentioned previously, one possible explanation for this could be that the child is allergic to elements other than caffeine in the chocolate and cola botanical family of food. Some hyperactive children calm down when given tea or coffee. (Many of my young patients were on Ritalin or other stimulant medication, which they took before breakfast and lunch, but

after school a cup of tea did the trick.) On the other hand, some children become wired by even small amounts of caffeine.

To test tea, use regular, not herbal tea. Some children like iced tea mixed with Minute Maid lemonade better than hot tea. Use regular coffee; again, some children like it cold.

Artificial Colors

To test artificial colors, purchase a set of Schilling Assorted Food Colors and Egg Dye. Each kit includes red, green, yellow and blue. Unfortunately, the list of chemicals used in the dyes is not included. To test yellow, you can add it to apple juice, lemonade and peach slurpees. Red can be added to stew, cranberry cocktail and raspberry or strawberry juice. Green can be added to limeade. Blue can be added to a fruit punch to make it look like grape punch.

To test tartrazine (yellow dye #5), you can use the following foods, provided your child is not intolerant of other ingredients in them: orange Tang, lime Gatorade, Kraft Golden Blend Italian Dressing, French's Seasoning Salt, Kraft Macaroni and Cheese Dinner*. Alpha Bits contain oat flour, sugar, pregelatinized corn flour, salt, honey, tartrazine, iron and B vitamins. This is a good cereal to use to test for tartrazine if corn and sugar are not a problem for your child.

You may wonder why it is important to test dyes. One of the main reasons is that many medications contain dyes. Most pediatric medications are a banquet of artificial colors and flavors. It is therefore important to know whether or not your child will tolerate them before you buy them.

Artificial Flavors

If you decided to test all artificial flavors, you would never finish. Among those recognized as problems by many

* At the time of writing all these products contained tartrazine.

parents are artificial maple, artificial vanilla, malt and caramel. Artificial maple can be found in pancake syrups other than pure maple syrup. Artificial vanilla extract is made by several companies. The chemical composition of malt and the amount of it contained in a product may vary from product to product. If your child reacts to Old Dutch Bavarian Pretzels, which contain only flour, salt, malt, yeast and sodium hydrate, you can safely assume that malt is the culprit if the other ingredients are tolerated. Post Grape Nuts contain only wheat, malted barley, salt, yeast, amylase, iron and vitamins. If tolerated, this is an excellent cereal and can make a good crunchy base for gorp. Some children react to caramel flavoring. Its chemical composition also varies from product to product. Since there is such a variety of ingredients in caramel, you will have to test each product containing it individually.

Spices

Some children are intolerant of certain spices. Having your child sniff the spice is a reasonable way of testing it. Another way to test it is to put it in something you are baking. The most common problem spices are nutmeg, ginger, cloves, cinnamon and, less often, turmeric, mustard and curry.

While teaching early childhood nutrition at a community college, I did an interesting experiment. The students were given ingredient listings for four packaged foods. They were asked to choose the two that they thought were nutritious versus the two that had little nutritional merit. When the results were tallied, I discovered that they all thought popular brands of cat and dog food had more nutritional value than popular brands of high-sugar cereal and corn munchies. No, they didn't start snacking on pet food, but they certainly were impressed! It is frightening to think that we feed our pets better than ourselves.

When making your decision about what to reintroduce into your child's diet, ask yourself:

- Is the product nutritious?
- Is it low in sugar?
- If it has additives, are the additives being used to enhance the product's appearance or to preserve it?
- If the additives are for preservative purposes, is there another similar preservative-free product that is reasonably priced?
- If it doesn't have preservatives, do I know the proper food handling and storage techniques?

It is not the end of the world if our children have an occasional empty calorie treat, but good parenting includes providing a nutritious, varied, low-additive diet garnished with hugs and kisses. As one mother said: "If someone had told me a change in diet was all it would take to improve family life, I would have snickered and eaten another chocolate chip cookie. But when it's proven to you that your child regularly goes into the twilight zone on that same chocolate chip cookie (and other foods), the decision to eat differently is easy. Naturally, it's not all that easy. I sometimes feel like a born-again hippie looking for additive-free ingredients, but the cooking is a breeze. As for Jamie, he doesn't get the food treats other kids do, but he sure enjoys the friendly attention that naturally goes to kids who stand still long enough to receive it."

ADAPTING MENUS
FOR OTHER FAMILY MEMBERS

ALTHOUGH THE Hyperactivity Test Diet menus have been designed to appeal to children, there is no reason that other family members cannot follow this diet or adapt it to their needs. Many parents have reported dramatic improvement in themselves on the diet—better sleep, decreased headaches and fewer gastrointestinal upsets.

There is little published scientific data to prove that the elimination of potential allergens and additives during pregnancy and breast-feeding will prevent poor behavior, sleep and physical symptoms in the newborn. However, in my clinical work, evidence certainly supports removing or restricting the foods and chemicals from the mother's diet which appear to cause problems for that particular family. I have seen fussy, miserable, gassy, tired, breast-fed babies become normal within seventy-two hours of mothers' removing food additives, stimulants and caffeine from their diets (even when the mothers had only been having minimal amounts of caffeine-containing foods). Occasionally, I have seen young babies' behavior improve dramatically when all scented products (popular brands of disposable diapers, baby lotions, parents' scented toiletries, room fresheners) are removed.

Seldom is there more than one hyperactive child in the family, though younger siblings tend to imitate older brothers and sisters. Often you will find one hyperactive, one asthmatic and perhaps another child with eczema all in the same family. Of course, no grown-up would admit to having behavioral problems, but they might confess to having a physical problem or a sleep problem. All family members could benefit from this diet.

NUTRIENT REQUIREMENTS

As MENTIONED IN Chapter 6, the meals for the diet have been carefully planned to provide all the needed nutrients (except calcium and vitamin D) for the average four-to six-year-old. If you want to adapt the diet for other members of your family or yourself, you should increase or decrease portion sizes, depending on the ages of the others. If you follow the diet, the only supplements you will require are calcium, which you should take on a daily basis, and vitamin D. The latter only needs to be taken during the winter months. If you become pregnant while on the diet, you should consult a dietitian. The menu plan as mapped out in the daily menus provides approximately 1500 calories or 6500 kJ a day.

The foods, menus and recipes provided in this book certainly should not be harmful to any members of the family unless one or more has food allergies or intolerances not taken into consideration by this plan. Outlined below are some substitutions you can make for items on the diet that some family members may not tolerate:

PEANUT BUTTER: I seriously considered removing peanut butter from the trial diet because some children very definitely have behavioral reactions to it. If other nuts are not a problem, other nut butters can be substituted. Otherwise, homemade sunflower or sesame butter can be substituted.

NUTS: Nuts are a big problem for some allergic people. Sesame seeds, sunflower seeds and pumpkin seeds make reasonable alternatives.

BUTTER: Some of the children that I have had on a similar diet are so sensitive to milk and dairy products that they are also intolerant of butter. If this is the case for your child, you might try Shedd's Willow Run Margarine on vegetables and main courses or substitute homemade mayonnaise, lemon juice, vinegar, homemade French dressing or fresh herbs for flavoring. For baking, use appropriate oils.

EGGS: A number of egg substitutes are available for baking. They are typically sold in small boxes which appear to be expensive, but a little bit goes a long way.

WHEAT: Wheat is definitely one of the more difficult items to remove from one's diet, and I strongly recommend that if you are put on a wheat-free trial, you engage the services of a dietitian to get you going. You will note that the product list gives suggestions for many non-wheat crackers and cereals. Chinese groceries normally have rice vermicelli, which you can use as a substitute for pasta. Again, the allergy cookbooks included in the Recommended Reading List, local allergy associations and local celiac associations offer many suggestions and recipes for wheat-free diets. Beware of the recipes for celiacs that call for wheat starch. If you have a wheat allergy, it is best to avoid wheat completely.

OTHER SPECIAL NEEDS

THIS DIET CAN BE easily adapted to meet other special needs, such as low cholesterol or low sodium requirements. This is because most of the foods and recipes the diet calls for have no hidden or special ingredients, and substitutions can be made easily. Older children and adults who have been advised to reduce their fat and salt intake can adapt this diet by eating more whole grain bread and cereals (include both oat and wheat bran) and fewer higher-fat cookies. They should also eat more fruit and vegetables and reduce the amount of nuts and seeds they eat that are high in fat. As well, they should decrease the amount of fats and oils called for in some recipes and omit salt altogether. If you have other special needs, it would be well worthwhile to consult a dietitian and have him or her help you make the necessary adaptations.

OTHER ADULT ADAPTATIONS

MOST OF MY ADULT FRIENDS who have tried the diet continue to consume copious quantities of tea and coffee and soft drinks that contain caffeine. If you fit into this category, unless you want to suffer from headaches, nausea, irritability and stomach upset, do not eliminate the tea, coffee and cola from your diet all at once. Most people who cut these things out overnight suffer miserable withdrawal symptoms, and it really isn't necessary. If you gradually reduce your intake by about one cup every two days, you should not suffer these symptoms. It might be best to go through this gradual elimination process before beginning the diet. On the other hand, if moderate amounts of tea and coffee do not bother you, there is no need to deprive yourself of these popular beverages. If you do decide to eliminate them from your diet, do be careful about selecting alternatives. Many herbal teas and coffee substitutes contain stimulants and ingredients that are restricted on this diet. A few of the herbal teas which may be acceptable are: rosehip, lemon balm, raspberry, strawberry and black currant. A suggested coffee substitute is Inka.

Most alcoholic beverages contain a gold mine of ingredients that are restricted on this diet. Why not give your liver a break and have a cool sparkling mineral water with a twist of lime?

FOOD PRODUCT LIST

AT THE TIME that this list was compiled, the following foods did not contain the additives and ingredients that are avoided on this diet. However, manufacturers can at any time change the ingredients of their products. Please continue to be a label reader.

Milk Substitutes:
Soy milk and soy milk powder; for example, Nutri-max, Vitasoy, limited amounts of coconut milk.

Butter:
Uncolored butter. Check with your local dairies. Often during the summer months, color is not added to butter. Some dairies will make you a special order of uncolored butter if you order a large amount.

Margarine:
Shedd's Willow Run Margarine (soy, water, Vitamin A, carotene, salt).

Ice Cream:
Soy frozen desserts are available in several areas. Check labels for suitability of ingredients. Or make homemade soy frozen desserts or fruit ices.

Peanut Butter:
Fresh ground peanut butter; Smuckers All Natural; Skippy Old-Fashioned (peanuts and salt); Adams Unsalted 100% Natural.

For variety try other nut butters, such as Roaster Fresh Cashew or Sunflower.

Fats and Oils:
For health reasons, choose polyunsaturated oil such as Wesson Sunflower Oil or pure monounsaturated oils such as Crisco Puritan Oil; pure olive oil. There are a variety of pure oils on the market without preservatives.

Eggs:
Any.

Breads:
When checking the suitability of its bread with a bakery, check that the bread contains: untreated flour, no malt or caramel, no milk or dairy products, no propionic acid or propionates. Also verify that the wrappers are not treated with BHT or BHA and that preservative-free oils have been used in the bread and to grease the pans. Bakeries will often make a special order of bread if you are prepared to buy approximately one to two dozen loaves.

Crackers:
Homemade melba toast; Ryvita Rye Crisp in white package; Ryvita Snackbread; Chico San Buckwheat or Sesame Rice Cakes; Quaker Rice Cakes (plain). There are many suitable puffed rice cakes available. Check labels. Kavli Norwegian Flatbread (rye flour, yeast, water, salt); Hol Grain Brown Rice Lite Snack Thins (rice, with and without salt); Wasa Light (rye flour, salt, water) and Golden Crackers (rye flour, yeast, salt and water).

Hot Cereal:

• Quick Quaker Oats; Quaker Whole Wheat Hot Natural Cereal; Cream of Wheat; Pure Oat Bran Cereals; American Home Food Products Wheatena (all natural);

- Heinz, Gerber or Mead Johnson Oatmeal Cereal; Mead Johnson or Gerber Rice Cereal. The malt in these infant cereals does not appear to cause a problem.
- Lifestream Rice Cream and Erewhon Brown Rice Cream. (These are not supplemented with iron as are the Heinz, Gerber and Mead Johnson infant cereals.)

Serve with fruit, puréed fruit, soy or coconut milk.

Cold Cereal:
Any plain puffed rice or wheat; all Health Valley puffed cereals except corn; Post Bran Flakes; Nature's Path Fiber O's (whole oat flour, brown rice flour, oat bran, concentrated pineapple, pear and peach juice). They make good munchies.

Unfortunately, many of the other natural, preservative-free cereals contain either corn or raisins.

Flour:
Many mills, including Arrowhead Mills have untreated flour. Store opened flour in a cool place. Store-brand bran and wheat germ are acceptable. Refrigerate opened wheat germ. Erewhon and Millstream carry a variety of untreated flours.

Rice:
Any plain white or brown rice.

Pasta:
DiCecco, Roma, Lancia, Catelli or health food varieties such as DeBole's. Some other brands contain yellow dye.

Bars and Cookies:
El Molino Graham Honey Animal Cookies (whole wheat flour, honey, soybean oil, oats, unsulphured molasses, lecithin, natural flavor, baking soda, wheat germ). Sev-

eral recipes for easy, homemade, low-sugar cookies are included in Chapter 7.

Meat, Fish and Poultry:

Any fresh or frozen plain beef, veal, lamb, pork, poultry, fish, game; Bumble Bee Alaska Pink Salmon or Star-Kist Tuna in Water; Carnation Baby Clams; Libby's Corned Beef. Read your labels.

Avoid self-basted turkeys and prestuffed meats. Some people who are sensitive to their environment react to meat which has been barbecued, especially on a charcoal barbecue. Smoked, pickled and processed meats should be excluded during this trial period unless you find a sausagemaker who will make ham, bacon or wieners with recommended ingredients.

Fruit:

Fruit is a natural source of sugar. Ideally it should be served at the end of a meal or with a high protein food.

All fresh fruits except apples, oranges and grapes are allowed. If fresh fruit is not available, use loosely packed frozen unsweetened fruit (blueberries, strawberries, raspberries, rhubarb and cherries are readily available). Use currants, dates or figs instead of raisins.

Choose unsweetened canned fruits in suitable juice or water, such as Dole Pineapple, DelMonte Fruit Naturals. Read labels. There are many brands available.

Fruit Juice:

Dilute all allowed juices fifty-fifty with water when using as a beverage. Whenever possible choose unsweetened pure juices. Choose canned, frozen or bottled juices. To increase variety, some presweetened juices have been included in the following list:

• Pineapple: a variety of canned and frozen unsweetened.
• Grapefruit: a variety of canned, bottled and frozen.

- Lemon: Minute Maid frozen.
- Lemonade: Minute Maid frozen (not pink).
- Limeade: Minute Maid frozen.
- Pear: Gerber Pear Juice from concentrate or use pear juice drained from canned fruit.
- Prune: Welch's Prune Nectar, bottled.
- Cranberry: Ocean Spray Cranberry Cocktail, bottled.

Ribena Black Currant, Kraus Cherry, Raspberry and Black Currant Fruit Syrups are very high in sugar, but a small amount added to sparkling water makes a great fruit pop.

Vegetables:
All fresh vegetables except tomatoes and corn are acceptable. Read labels on frozen plain vegetables and plain canned vegetables to ensure that they don't contain inappropriate additives.

Baking Supplies:

- Any baking powder or soda; cream of tartar.
- Sweeteners: in moderation, white or brown sugar
  Pure maple syrup: Cary's Maple Syrup
  Syrup: Lyle's Golden (100% cane), Tree Brand
  Molasses: Canasoy Unsulphured, Crosby's Pure.
- Salt and pepper, paprika, bay leaves, celery seed.
- Fresh garlic, pure garlic powder.
- All green herbs, dill weed and seed.
- McCormick Italian Seasoning (marjoram, thyme, rosemary, savory, sage, oregano, sweet basil).
- Spices: cinnamon, cumin, coriander, allspice, fennel, anise, ginger. DO NOT USE cloves, nutmeg, curry and turmeric.
- Pure vanilla extract or bean: If your child has an alcohol intolerance, do not use the extract. Instead make vanilla sugar by mixing (2 cups) 500 mL white sugar with a 1-

inch vanilla bean; keep in a screw-top jar for two weeks
before using.
- Pure carob powder as a substitute for chocolate. Milk-
free carob chips are available in specialty shops.
- Baking yeast: any brand.
- Davis or Knox Unflavored Gelatin. (Gelatin added to
homemade popsicles keeps them from dripping.)
- Unsweetened coconut, dried figs, dates, apricots, currants, papaya, pineapple.
- Plain nuts (available in the baking section of the store
rather than the snack section); plain sunflower and sesame seeds.
- Plain white vinegar. (Make herbal vinegars for variety.)

Condiments and Jams:

- Homemade mayonnaise and salad dressings.
- Tamari Soya Sauce.
- Homemade rhubarb ketchup, zucchini relish and mus-
tard.
- Any pure honey in moderation.
- Pure jam made with allowed fruits in moderation; for
example, Kraft Pure Raspberry, Strawberry, Apricot,
Red Currant, Peach; Smuckers Seedless Strawberry
Jam, Red Rasberry Preserves, and Currant Jelly.

Treats:

- Potato chips: Old Fashioned Kettle Cooked Cape Cod,
FritoLay's Ruffles.
- Sesame snacks in moderation.
- Peanuts and nuts in the shell; plain nuts and seeds can
be toasted in the oven and salted.
- Sorbee Natural Sugarless Pops, lemon and lime, for
treats in moderation. They contain sorbitol and may
cause diarrhea if eaten excessively.
- Gummy bears in moderation (gelatin, fruit juice, glu-

cose, citric acid). Read labels as there are gummy bears made with artificial color and flavor. The real ones are expensive.

Beverages:

- Sparkling or natural mineral water. There are many suitable brands, such as Canada Dry or Perrier. Read labels. Some may have benzoates.
- A small scoop of pure frozen juice concentrate added to sparkling water makes an excellent fruit pop.
- Regular 7Up in moderation or fifty-fifty mix with sparkling water.
- Adults using a modified version of this diet plan may want to substitute herbal teas for tea and coffee: pure rosehip, strawberry, black currant, lemon balm, linden. Coffee substitute: Krakus Inka (roasted barley, rye, chicory, beet roots).

APPENDIX C

Non-Food Product List

In addition to having food allergies, some hyperactive children have intolerances to non-food items, such as air fresheners and other scented products. No one really needs to use these products, and we are certainly doing our allergic friends a favor if we can invite them to an unscented home. The following suggested products are by no means all those available, but they are products used by many families.

Unscented/Low Scent Soap:
Ivory, Jergens La Palina Castile, Aveeno (oatmeal-based), White Palmolive, Dove Unscented Beauty Bar, Pure and Natural.

Toothpaste:
Baking soda and/or salt are probably the safest substitute. If you must use a regular toothpaste, choose a white toothpaste, not a gel or striped paste.

Fluoride:
Drops or pills if water in your area is not fluoridated. There is an unflavored gel for fluoride treatment, which you can get from your dentist.

Shampoo and Hair Conditioner:
Choose unscented, such as Ivory Free Unscented Shampoo and Conditioner.

Skin Lotion:
pHisoderm Unscented Skin Cleaner and Conditioner.

Deodorants:
Unscented white, such as Arrid Extra Dry Solid Unscented, Soft & Dri Solid Unscented.

Lip Gloss and Mascara:
Substitute Vaseline.

Cosmetics:
Choose an unscented hypoallergenic brand that is right for you: Marcelle, Clinique, Almay, Jaffra, Aziza. Many of my allergic patients tolerate cosmetics better if they alternate them.

Hairspray:
Clairol Final Net Unscented (pump), Non-Aerosol Silkience, Aqua-Net Unscented Hairspray (pump).

Disposable Diapers:
Huggies, Luvs. Sears also has unscented disposable diapers. If you are concerned about our environment, cloth diapers (home-laundered or from a diaper service) are a much better choice.

Room Deodorizers:
Burning a wooden match removes odors, as does opening a window. A dish of charcoal briquets or vinegar makes a good odor eater. To get rid of odors in your refrigerator, place an open box of baking soda in it. For a pleasant scent, gently simmer tolerated herbs or spices in water on the stove.

Cleaning Supplies:

• Vinegar, 1 tbsp (15 mL) per quart (liter) of water for light cleaning

- Arm & Hammer Washing Soda
- Borax
- Bon Ami
- Olive oil on a cloth for polishing wooden furniture
- Oxydol or Unscented Tide Laundry Detergent
- Woolite Gentle Laundry Detergent
- Clorox II Bleach
- Ivory Liquid Dish Detergent
- Cascade or Electrasol Dishwasher Detergent
- Cheer Free Liquid Laundry Detergent
- Ivory Snow Laundry Soap Flakes

Water:

Occasionally, the chlorine in drinking water and water for general use, as well as in swimming pool water, poses a problem. If your child is only slightly intolerant of chlorine, a thorough shower with soap immediately after using a swimming pool should be adequate. If the intolerance is more severe, thiosulphate (available in pet stores) can be added to bath water to change chlorine to chloride.

Water purifiers can be purchased which remove chlorine and other undesirables from water but leave the minerals intact.

Paper Goods:

Use white unscented tissues and toilet paper, and white paper towels, serviettes and cupcake liners.

Toys and Art Supplies:

Check these children's play supplies for suitability: playdough, finger paints, watercolors, felt and ball point pens, scratch and sniff books, Silly Putty, colored Tinker-Toy sticks, powder in balloons, colored chalk and chalk dust, food for play ovens and dolls. If the item in question smells or the color comes off, be suspicious. If new toys, such as some plastic dolls, emit a strange smell, give them a couple of soapy baths and dry them out of doors in the sunshine.

Some suitable school supplies are:

- Flo Marker (Faber Castell)
- Faber Castell Textliners
- Vis-a-Vis Broad Tip Pens
- Crayola Markers (not fruit-scented)
- Bic Crayons (felt tip)
- Jiffy Water Soluble Fibre Tip Pens
- Elmer's Mucilage Glue
- Taperaser Correction Fluid

Even though these products are safe, the child should wash his or her hands well after using them as an extra precaution.

Household Products and Other Environmental Factors to Watch out for:
Cigarette smoke, gas and oil, lead, insect sprays, tar, artificial lighting, paint/varnish, newsprint, scented candles, incense, mothballs, scented pads and tampons. By becoming more aware of scents, you will be able to determine whether or not they are a problem for your family.

ALLERGY ASSOCIATIONS

Allergy:

Allergy Information, P.O. Box 640, Menlo Park, CA. 94026. Tel. (415) 322-1663. Recorded message advises that the organization provides allergy information by mail. Send a self addressed envelope and two stamps.

Asthma and Allergy Foundation of America, 1302 18th Street, N.W. Suite 303, Washington, D.C. 20036. Tel. (202) 293-2950. Highly recommended by both professionals and parents for providing excellent information and educational materials to the public.

The National Allergy and Asthma Network, 3554 Chain Bridge Road, Suite 200, Fairfax, Va. 22030 Tel. 703-385-4403 or 4404. Dynamic parent-driven organization offers a monthly, 8 page newsletter and a variety of resources including: videos, books and pamphlets.

The National Institute of Allergy and Infectious Diseases, Building 31, Room 7 A 32, 9000 Rockville Pike, Bethesda, Md. 20205. The institute is known for good professional information. Some lay publications are available.

The Allergy Information Association, 65 Tromley Drive, Suite 10, Islington, Ontario, Canada, M9B 5Y7 Tel. (416) 244-8585. This well established association has a large American membership and offers an excellent quarterly newsletter and frequently updated information sheets.

Diet and Behavior:

The Feingold Association of the United States, Box 6550, Alexandria, VA 22306 Tel. (703) 768-FAUS. The program promoted by this group is based on a diet eliminating synthetic colors, synthetic flavors, the preservatives BHT, BHA and TBHQ. Natural salicylates and aspirin are initially removed and subsequently reintroduced if they do not cause reactions. Although the Feingold Diet, instructions for use, reintroduction of foods and theory, differ from some of the information presented in this book, the group offers excellent, compatible publications including:

Food List (for different areas in the United States)

Medication List

Recipes (especially useful for a salicylate intolerance)

If using these publications, it is very important to continue to read labels carefully, as many foods acceptable on a Feingold diet may contain ingredients not acceptable on this test diet e.g. milk and dairy products, MSG, HVP, HPP, caffeine.

It is suggested that parents contact their local hospitals, child development centers, and schools for information about local support groups, appropriate parenting courses and allergy information groups.

RECOMMENDED READING

General:

Child of Mine—Feeding with Love and Good Sense, Expanded edition, Ellyn Satter R.D. (Bull Publishing Co. Palo Alto, CA, 1986). Excellent, up-to-date, easy to read book on feeding—from pregnancy through the toddler period. The book focuses on parenting/feeding techniques and is a must for parents experiencing difficulties feeding their young children.

How to Get Your Child to Eat . . . But Not too Much, Ellyn Satter R.D. (Bull Publishing Co. Palo Alto, CA, 1987). This practical, book addresses parenting/feeding techniques from birth through adolescence. Of special interest for parents with allergic or food intolerant children and/or children with developmental disabilities are the chapters on feeding the child who grows poorly and feeding the child with special needs.

Allergy and Food Intolerance Information:

Coping with Food Allergy, Claude A. Frazier (Quadrangle Books, New York, 1985). A good resource book for parents and professionals.

In Bad Taste The MSG Syndrome, George Schwartz (Signet, New York, 1988). A must for people with an intolerance to monosodium glutamate. The book includes lists of brand-name products containing MSG, misleading labeling information, as well as clinical case studies and symptoms of intolerance.

149

Attention Deficit Disorder or Hyperactivity:

Understanding and Managing Overactive Children, Don H. Fontenelle (Prentice-Hall, New Jersey, 1983). This easy to read book discusses all causes of and treatments for overactive children. Professional colleagues, experienced with support groups and families with hyperactive children, have highly recommended this book. The chapter on diet and nutrition describes the two therapies/theories popular at the time of publication.

SELECTED REFERENCES

Material from the following sources was of the utmost value in the writing of this book.

Benton, D., and Roberts, G. "Effect of vitamin and mineral supplementation on intelligence of a sample of school children." *Lancet* 23 Jan. 1988: 140-143.

Brostoff, J., and Challacombe, S.J. *Food Allergy and Intolerance.* London, England: Ballière Tindall, 1987.

Butkus, S.N., and Mahan, L.K. "Food Allergies: immunological reactions to food." *Journal of the American Dietetic Association* 86 (1986): 601-608.

Collins-Williams, C. "Clinical spectrum of adverse reactions to tartrazine." *Journal of Asthma* 22 (1985): 139-143.

Egger, J. "Food allergy and the central nervous system." In *Food Allergy, Nestlé Nutrition Workshop Series* 17. Raven Press, 1988: 159-175.

Egger, J.; Carter, C.M.; Soothill, J.F.; Wilson, J. "Oligoantigenic diet treatment of children with epilepsy and migraine." *Journal of Pediatrics* 114 (1989): 51-55.

Egger, J.; Graham, P.J.; Carter, C.M.; Gumly, D.; Soothill, J.F. "Controlled trial of oligoantigenic treatment in the hyperactive syndrome." *Lancet,* 9 March 1985: 540-545.

Feingold, B. *Why Your Child Is Hyperactive.* New York: Random House, 1976.

Goyette, C.H.; Conners, C.K.; Ulrich, R.F. "Normative data on revised Conners parent and teacher rating scales." *Journal of Abnormal Child Psychology* 6 (1978): 221-236.

Jenkins et al. "Glycemic Index." *American Journal of Clinical*

Nutrition 34 (1981): 362-366.

Kaplan, B.J., "The Relevance of food for children's cognitive and behavioral health." *Canadian Journal of Behavioral Science* 20 (1988): 359-373.

Kaplan, B.J.; McNicol, J.; Conte, R.A.; Moghadam, H.K. "Sleep disturbances in preschool-aged hyperactive and normal children." *Pediatrics* 80 (1987): 839-844.
—"Physical signs and symptoms in preschool-aged hyperactive and normal children." *Journal of Developmental and Behavioral Pediatrics* 8 (1987): 305-310.
—"Dietary replacement in preschool-aged hyperactive boys." *Pediatrics* 83 (1989): 7-17.
—"Overall nutrient intake of preschool hyperactive and normal boys." *Journal of Abnormal Child Psychology* 17 (1989): 127-132.
—"Nutrient intakes of preschool-aged boys." *Journal of the Canadian Dietetic Association* 50 (1989): 31-35.

The NUTS Nutrition Assessment System, Version 3.3, 1987. Victoria, B.C.: Quilchena Consulting Ltd.

Rowe, K.S. "Synthetic food colourings and 'hyperactivity': A double-blind crossover study." *Australian Paediatrics Journal* 24 (1988): 143-147.

Small, B.M. et al. *Recommendations for Action on Pollution and Education in Toronto.* Consultation paper prepared for the Toronto Board of Education, Toronto, Ontario, 1985.

RECIPE INDEX

SUBJECT INDEX

157